DRESDEN TEAMWORK CONCEPT FOR MEDICAL HIGH RISK ORGANIZATIONS

DRESDEN TEAMWORK CONCEPT FOR MEDICAL HIGH RISK ORGANIZATIONS

AXEL R. HELLER
EDITOR

Nova Science Publishers, Inc.
New York

For permission to use material from this book please contact us:
Telephone 631-231-7269; Fax 631-231-8175
Web Site: http://www.novapublishers.com

NOTICE TO THE READER

The Publisher has taken reasonable care in the preparation of this book, but makes no expressed or implied warranty of any kind and assumes no responsibility for any errors or omissions. No liability is assumed for incidental or consequential damages in connection with or arising out of information contained in this book. The Publisher shall not be liable for any special, consequential, or exemplary damages resulting, in whole or in part, from the readers' use of, or reliance upon, this material. Any parts of this book based on government reports are so indicated and copyright is claimed for those parts to the extent applicable to compilations of such works.

Independent verification should be sought for any data, advice or recommendations contained in this book. In addition, no responsibility is assumed by the publisher for any injury and/or damage to persons or property arising from any methods, products, instructions, ideas or otherwise contained in this publication.

This publication is designed to provide accurate and authoritative information with regard to the subject matter covered herein. It is sold with the clear understanding that the Publisher is not engaged in rendering legal or any other professional services. If legal or any other expert assistance is required, the services of a competent person should be sought. FROM A DECLARATION OF PARTICIPANTS JOINTLY ADOPTED BY A COMMITTEE OF THE AMERICAN BAR ASSOCIATION AND A COMMITTEE OF PUBLISHERS.

LIBRARY OF CONGRESS CATALOGING-IN-PUBLICATION DATA
Heller, Axel R.
  Dresden teamwork concept for medical high risk organizations / Axel R. Heller.
     p. ; cm.
  Includes bibliographical references and index.
  ISBN 978-1-60692-307-8 (hardcover)
  1. Hospitals--Risk management. 2. Hospitals--Quality control. 3. Hospitals--Administration. 4. Health care teams. I. Title. II. Title: Teamwork concept for medical high risk organizations.
  [DNLM: 1. Technische Universität Dresden. Universitätsklinikum. 2. Risk Management--methods. 3. Hospital Administration. 4. Institutional Management Teams. 5. Quality Assurance, Health Care. WX 157 H4765d 2009]
  RA971.38.H47 2009
  362.11068--dc22   2008039816

Published by Nova Science Publishers, Inc. ✦ *New York*

CONTENTS

PREFACE

Besides its core competencies in excellent patient care the university hospital Dresden Germany focuses on team- and quality management. In our understanding team management is one key success factor for hospitals in the future.

Excellent nationally and internationally recognized projects and practice proven concepts will be presented by specialists in their fields. After discussing the strategic background and advantages of team oriented management from the hospital CEOs viewpoint, possibilities of aligning individual employee performance with strategic goals under the peculiarities of university hospitals are presented. The concept of shared mental models is then closely discussed on the background of cutting edge results in this field in a guest article by Piet van den Bossche (Dept. of Educational development and Educational Research, Maastricht University/ The Netherlands). Fitting just into the latter empirical background, team concepts in Helicopter Emergency Medical Services are described, which rely on shared mental models of all team members. To achieve good Crew Resource Management the Dresden Six Step Approach of CRM improves team performance by introducing psychological know how into simulator based teaching focusing on shared mental models and team effectiveness.

The next chain link of patient safety is risk management representing a vital part of quality management in high risk medical organizations. In this regard the design and implementation of a local Critical Incident Reporting System (CIRS) in Dresden is illustrated. Consequently the results of our CIRS are openly discussed as well as the changes in daily practice derived from its reports. The next step on the way to business excellence is the utilization of closed quality management circuits referring to the classical Deming cycle (plan- do- check- act). In this regard the authors describe the results of the first Six Sigma team optimization project in a German hospital in collaboration with the Chair of Market oriented Corporate Management and Marketing of the University of Dresden.

Responsibility for society is further taken by setting up a quality certified a transregional stroke management network. Using virtual patient gateways under the leadership of the UHD quality in patient care evolves from the local level of one hospital to the entire eastern Saxon region. Most fascinating and challenging, however is psychology and team management of large teams and resources under time pressure exemplified in mass casualty incidents and natural disasters directly affecting a level 3 trauma center as illustrated in the both final chapters.

This book is aimed to managers and team leaders, practitioners, and team members in diverse organizations as well as management consultants. This diverse target group illustrates the basic approach of team management. Only the strategy oriented inter-professional coop-eration of management and staff within shared mental models across the organization enables sustained success of all contributors lastly by increasing patient safety and satisfaction.

Chapter 1

INTRODUCTION: MANAGING HUMAN RESOURCES IN MEDICAL HIGH RISK ORGANIZATIONS

Axel R. Heller

Dept. Anesthesiology and Intensive care Medicine
University Hospital Carl Gustav Carus
University of Technology, Dresden, Germany

SUMMARY

Besides its core competencies in excellent patient care the university hospital Dresden Germany focuses on team- and quality management. In our understanding team management is one key success factor for hospitals in the future.

Excellent nationally and internationally recognized projects and practice proven concepts will be presented by specialists in their fields. After discussing the strategic background and advantages of team oriented management from the hospital CEOs viewpoint, possibilities of aligning individual employee performance with strategic goals under the peculiarities of university hospitals are presented. The concept of shared mental models is then closely discussed on the background of cutting edge results in this field in a guest article by Piet van den Bossche (Dept. of Educational development and Educational Research, Maastricht University/ The Netherlands). Fitting just into the latter empirical background, team concepts in Helicopter Emergency Medical Services are described, which rely on shared mental models of all team members. To achieve good Crew Resource Management the Dresden Six Step Approach of CRM improves team performance by introducing psychological know how into simulator based teaching focusing on shared mental models and team effectiveness.

The next chain link of patient safety is risk management representing a vital part of quality management in high risk medical organizations. In this regard the design and implementation of a local Critical Incident Reporting System (CIRS) in Dresden is illustrated. Consequently the results of our CIRS are openly discussed as well as the changes in daily practice derived from its reports. The next step on the way to business excellence is the utilization of closed quality management circuits referring to the classical Deming cycle (plan- do- check- act). In this regard we describe the results of the first Six Sigma team optimization project in a German hospital in collaboration with the Chair of Corporate Management and Marketing of the University of Dresden.

Responsibility for society is further taken by setting up a quality certified a trans-regional stroke management network. Using virtual patient gateways under the leadership of the UHD quality in patient care evolves from the local level of one hospital to the entire eastern Saxon region. Most fascinating and challenging, however is psychology and team management of large teams and resources under time pressure exemplified in mass casualty incidents and natural disasters directly affecting a level 3 trauma center as illustrated in the both final chapters.

This book is aimed to managers and team leaders, practitioners, and team members in diverse organizations as well as management consultants. This diverse target group illustrates the basic approach of team management. Only the strategy oriented inter-professional cooperation of management and staff within shared mental models across the organization enables sustained success of all contributors lastly by increasing patient safety and satisfaction.

ENVIRONMENTAL CONSIDERATIONS

Problems of business structures also present in hospitals were pointed out by Bleicher [1] as follows: *"We work within **yesterdays** organizational structures using **today's** methods for **tomorrows** problems, largely with individuals having built **yesterdays** structures and who will not anymore experience **tomorrow** within the organization"*. Consequently these structures are neither adapted to the customers/ patients nor to the enablers of the system being represented by the processes and the employees [2]. Hence, **German health care institutions are widely not prepared for a competitive health care market** as proposed by implementation of a diagnoses related reimbursement system [3] paying the same compensation for the same procedure across the country. This problem will even get worse when pay for performance compensation will be introduced as already advocated in the US. **Advanced economic and staff leadership know how must, thus, be concern of all process participants in the hospital**. In this context excellent medical task management must be taken for granted as outlined in chapter two as future key factor of success in hospitals by Prof. D. Michael Albrecht M.D., the CEO of the University Hospital of Dresden (UHD). The earlier the organization is penetrated by a **spirit of service, quality and patient satisfaction** the higher is the competitive advantage. In this regard the work of the **middle management** [4] **must be aligned to the strategic goals of the hospital** and second must be phased which each other. This may be achieved using management by objectives as further discussed in chapter three, and by a leadership circle of the middle management (Führungskreis II/ FK II) to facilitate communication and to implement sustained strategy driven process orientation. The emotional effect has, likewise, to be taken into account and going a flexible "living example" by the top management is essential.

Regarding the environment of their jobs and assignments, the requirements of employees have emerged and nowadays they **claim for a new quality of thinking and acting in staff management**. Process related thinking and a respective understanding of roles is expected, characterized by **meaning, leeway, and fun** [5]. Thus, rationalistic leadership based on facts and figures has to be well balanced against emotional intelligence [6] founded in visions and moral values. In particular when economic pressure on medical high risk organizations increases, conflicting goals may occur and, thus, demand for new ways of management.

This book is aimed to team- leaders and managers in all areas, essentially contributing to creation of value in their organizations, open to think and act in new ways of leadership. In this regard managers and team leaders, practitioners, and team members of high risk-, health-care-, or business organizations are addressed. This **diverse target group** illustrates the **basic approach of team management**. Only the strategy **oriented inter-professional cooperation** of management and staff within **shared mental models across the organization** enables sustained success of all contributors lastly by increasing patient safety and satisfaction.

GOALS AND STRUCTURE OF THE BOOK

The exploration design for the Dresden teamwork activities (Figure 1) characterizes the structure and the arrangement of this book as well as the aims of the individual chapters. The x-axis represents the dimension of space starting with projects localized within the inner campus of UHD (local) up to exhaustive trans regional operations (right side). Additionally the figure distinguishes between a descriptive and a analytical view. The chapters above the space scale are descriptive, while the chapters below the x-axis are oriented analytically.

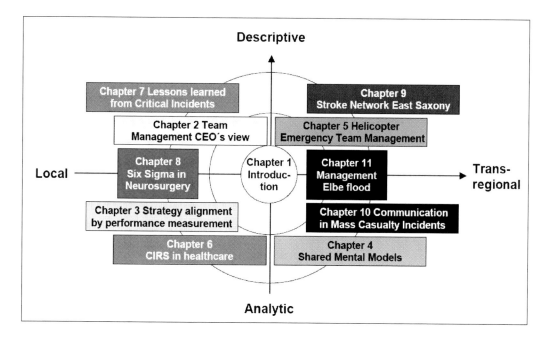

Figure 1. Exploration design and concept of the book.

The structure of the book and the orientation of the individual chapters may, thus, easily be comprehended. Following the introducing remarks chapters 2 and 3 describe internal (local) strategies of the UHD represented by concrete strategic positioning of the UHD within the current political environment including team leadership considerations on the level of top management (chapter 2) and by ways of strategy alignment from a more analytic point of view (chapter 3). The major problem of business management, also present in healthcare organizations, is to align the employees´ workforce with the companies strategy as well as with the long term goals of the top management [4]. Management by objectives (MbO) in this regard is the key link between the companies' strategy, individual assignments, and performance [7]. Chapter 3 besides general backgrounds on MbO discusses efforts and utility of performance measurement systems and incentives. Time and money spent for performance measurement systems, however, must clearly be weighed against improvement of corporate performance and key figures used must, undoubtedly, indicate what is intended to measure [8]. Overall, MbO bear the chance to improve the companies´ success to the degree individual salary is tied to the individuals contribution, lastly implementing entrepreneur way of thinking within each individual employee in the whole organization. To assure maximum achievement of companies goals, individual objectives and incentives have to be **distributed equitable** internally, **adjusted to corporate success, and to labor marked**. Most critical, however, is **horizontal adjustment of the stakeholders´ goals** across the organization.

The guest chapter 4 by Piet van den Bossche and co-workers from the Department of Educational Development and Educational Research, Faculty of Economics and Business Administration, Maastricht University, Netherlands, focuses on the experimental and theoretical background of shared mental models. This group over the last decade shed light on the limited understanding of the consequences of communication, team learning, and team-work for team performance and patient safety [9]. Empirical study data from team research in aviation or business provide enhanced understanding on how multi-professional teams interact socially, develop shared mental models determining cognitive performance as basis for sustained team success. Consequently they recommend that the field of **medicine must establish more attention to team processes with input from** research on **crew resource management** (CRM) in aviation, and team processes in business. But this requires the willingness of health care professionals to adapt these insights and modify them for their own professional context.

THE CHAIN OF PATIENT RISK

The chain of patient risk starts with fulfilling a certain risk of daily life and, consequently, turning a hazard into a real accident. Risk management in individual daily life consists of **bearing** or in some instances **insuring the risk**. These aspects of risk management are not in the focus of this book. Rather, risk **reduction and avoiding strategies** as utilized in the UHD are described. Figure 2, likewise, demonstrates the problem of accumulation of risks. Even if the risk e.g., death as a consequence of a single service as anesthesia is as low as death by a railroad incident (~1:500,000), the risk exponentially increases with the number of services applied. The **cumulative safety of a system** can be calculated as:

$$\text{Safety of single service}^{\text{number of services}}$$

Consequently, when 15 services are applied to one patient with a safety of 95% each, a cumulative safety of $0.95^{15} = 46\%$ results. From the calculatory point of view both, reduction of services involved e.g., by workflow standardization and increase in single service quality reduce the likelihood for the patient experiencing a undesired event. Following the incident the next chain links of patient risk subsequently are the Emergency Medical Service (EMS) and training methods addressed in chapter 5, anesthesia (chapter 6&7), and surgery itself (chapter 8).

The transfer of CRM to EMS as demanded in chapter 4 was done by Michael P. Müller M.D., who is the Head of the Dresden Interdisciplinary Simulator Center (ISIMED). In Helicopter Emergency Medical Services (HEMS) the problem of establishing shared mental models in **dynamic high risk environment** is exemplified within a **multidisciplinary team** under **time pressure**. **Dynamic decision making** is one of the key skills in crew resource management training in aviation [7]. In emergency medicine it is, likewise, important to practice this skill as a prerequisite for effective treatment of patients. In Germany HEMS represent the highest level of emergency treatment know how, thus HEMS is assigned to the most complex situations, even when ground EMS are already on site.

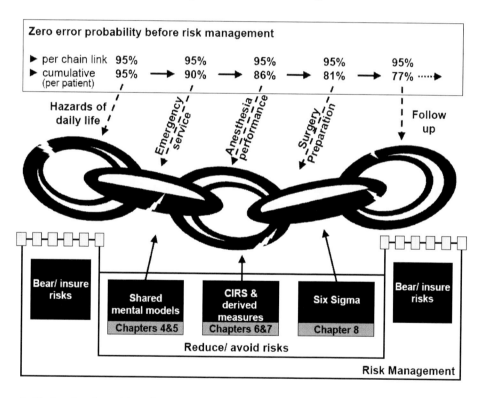

Figure 2: Chain of patient risk and examples of risk management strategies. Zero error probability in this figure was set to 95% (actually higher) to exemplify the effects on cumulative risk. Critical Incident Reporting System (CIRS)

During the pre-hospital treatment with limited diagnostic and therapeutic resources the patient's state has to be tracked continuously requiring repeated re-evaluation, because rapid change of patients' condition may occur. During the HEMS rescue mission initial therapeutic goals have, hence, dynamically to be adapted to current needs [10;11]. Likewise, tactical and technical tasks have to be managed by the multidisciplinary team consisting of one emergency physician who is defined as a *"medical passenger"* and not as flight crew member, one paramedic and one pilot, each experts in a extremely specialized area. Such problems are most complex, because a **multitude of information has to be processed and communicated across professional boundaries increasing the risk of overloading the human control span** [12]. With regard to cognition psychology a successful strategy requires **data reduction** to enable **sequential handling of single data packages** (see also Chapters 10 & 11). To achieve good Crew Resource Management (CRM) the Dresden Six Step Approach is described improving team performance by introducing psychological know how into CRM focusing on shared mental models and team effectiveness.

It is an open secret that medical services sometimes not only fail to improve patients but also cause avoidable damage. In a analytical way Matthias Hübler M.D., who is team leader of the Dresden Risk Management group and FK II member, addresses problems of the widespread **blame and shame culture** and how to implement a **local Critical Incident Reporting System** (CIRS) in chapter 6. The first step, however, must be the recognition that patient safety is a key factor to improve quality of healthcare organizations. In this context the most frustrating aspect is the apparent **failure of health-care systems to learn from their mistakes**. Too often health-care organizations ignore mishaps and hesitate to share information when an investigation has been carried out following an incident. As a consequence, the same mistakes occur repeatedly in many settings and patients continue to be harmed by preventable errors. Thus, reliable information about flaws in the treatment course must be gathered. This can be achieved by different means. One systematic way of collecting data is implementing a CIRS guaranteeing that the reporting person gets the **opportunity to communicate critical incidents without fearing negative personal consequences** and that the **information is shared** within the department or institution. A work group should **analyze the critical incident reports** on a **regular base** using **standardized protocols**. Focus should be set on organizational factors, which induced, aggravated or negatively influenced the adverse event or its seriousness rather than on personal factors. Finally, **consequences derived from reports should be made public** to improve quality and to increase the willingness to report.

Chapter 7 by Angela Möllemann M.D. who was part of a task force establishing a nationwide CIRS in Germany (www.pasos-ains.de) and who was deputy head of the Dresden risk management group describes the results and the lessons learned from risk management in the Dresden anesthesia department. 162 anonymous reports were received during a observation period of 18 months during which approximately 30.000 anesthesia procedures were performed. Messages showed a relative **overweight of vital emergency surgery insinuating a higher hazard likelihood**. The main causes were **distraction, lack of experience, specific training and communication deficits**. The confidence in the anonymity of the reporting system was very high. Following the analysis of the reports, several revisions of the workflow were implemented, e.g., definition of standards or specific training programs. This requires the **development of individual and institutional culture of dealing with error** and derived measures should be focused on training, technical modifications, definition or improvement/ adaptation of standards as well as in communication and teamwork training just in line with chapters 4 & 5.

The next step on the way to **business excellence** is the utilization of closed quality management circuits referring to the classical **Deming cycle (plan- do- check- act)** [13] and its further developments [14]. Staying on the local level of one Department in the UHD (Figure 1) Stephan B. Sobottka M.D. senior physician in Neurosurgery and FK II member together with co- workers from the Chair of Corporate Management an Marketing, University of

Dresden describes the adaption of the Six sigma concept, first invented by Motorola in 1987, to high risk medical processes in a both descriptive and analytical manner. The Six Sigma principle utilizes strategies, which are based on **quantitative measurements** and which seek to **optimize processes**, **limit deviations** or dispersion **from the target process**. Hence, Six Sigma aims to eliminate errors or quality problems. Therefore, **quality management tools are combined with advanced data analysis and systematic training of staff**. For the first time in German health system a pilot project to optimize the preparation for neurosurgical procedures could now show that using the Six Sigma method enhanced patient safety in medical care, while at the same time disturbances in the hospital processes could be avoided. Hence, the financial performance of the clinic was improved. The additional economic benefits of poorly quantifiable effects, such as the reduction of failure costs by avoided human and physical resources required for troubleshooting, future case number increases through enlarged satisfaction of patients, relatives, referring doctors and medical insurances or dropping liability insurance premiums/ avoided liability claims, were not evaluated in the project, however, the latter effects increase the economic advantage in favor of the clinic. With this chapter the description local quality management projects is completed and far reaching concepts addressing the society responsibilities of the UHD (Figure 1 right side) are presented.

TRANS-REGIONAL RESPONSIBILITIES OF THE UHD

Within rural East Saxony with approx. 1,600,000 citizens and additional 500,000 citizens in the capital of Dresden, the UHD is one of two level 3 trauma centers. Due to various factors (rural structures, demographics, salaries, brain drain) structure quality of the health care system in rural areas in former eastern Germany do not cover the actual demands [15]. To fight this structural problem, establishment of cooperation and networks across healthcare services and organizations care has been recognized as crucial. A major project by the German Federal Ministry of Education and Research termed "Health regions of the future" was set out to support five projects in Germany. A comprehensive project with more than 100 partner organizations under the leadership of the UHD named "Carus Consilium Sachsen" has made its way to the final assessment of the best 20 applications of more than 250 submitted. We are optimistic to succeed with our concept within this national competition.

The trans- regional project described in chapter 9 by Prof. Georg Gahn, M.D. vice head of the Department of Neurology UHD and former speaker of FK II will be one core project of "Carus Consilium Sachsen". He established a **widespread quality assured acute stroke care network** in the east Saxony rural area (Stroke-East-Saxony Network - SOS-NET) for patients, otherwise not having access to this type of care due to of **long distances to stroke units**. Thus, specialized treatment of stroke in general hospitals outside Dresden is supported by cooperation between the comprehensive UHD stroke center (CSC) and several affiliated general hospitals). Acute stroke therapy in the affiliated hospitals is guided through a VPN tunneled video and data conference. Quality assurance within the CSC and five satellite hospitals is based upon the ISO 9001:2000 quality management system and the requirements of the German Stroke Association. Tele-consultation and transfer of quality standards to the network partners improve patients´ outcome and reduces financial burdens of the health care system [16]. Besides considerations of patient care, tele-consultation for acute stroke therapy represents a spectacular tool for patient management which can be easily used as a marketing initiative by competing hospitals and, therefore to be an attractive extension to the hospitals´ service portfolios.

The escalation of the **imbalance between the need for healthcare services and its capacity** as previously described for rural areas in eastern Germany is, likewise, a hallmark of disaster medicine [17]. In particular multidisciplinary communication activities during mass casualty incidents are double edged because they must be subordinated under the major goal of mental model alignment of all participants to implement a **joint strategy under time pressure** [18]. In chapter 10 we analyze the way of team management and communication assuring proper accomplishment of the rescue mission. In the early stages of a mass casualty incident tactical **relevant information has to be filtered from a flood of data while organizational structure of emergency support is only slowly growing up**. Implementing organizational structure and subsidiary leadership within subunits [18] increases global efficacy by reducing tactical communication to a minimum. As in modern business management the organizational structure must follow the process which itself is determined by strategy [19]. Further a **unified management culture across all emergency management organizations and agencies by a joint leadership manual** focusing on the establishing a functional global organization facilitates timely implementation.

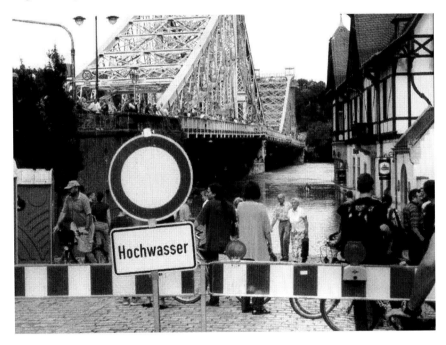

Figure 3. Thursday, 08/15/2002 at 2 p.m. Elbe floods at the river crossing "Blaues Wunder" built in 1893 (water level 8.9m (2m normal)). The worst case scenario was the tilt of this bridge, causing flash-flooding of the nearby University Hospital of Dresden © A. Heller..

The latter considerations were in particular challenged by the Elbe floods in 2002 as described in chapter 11, not only affecting one single hospital but the whole area demanding for trans regional rescue and team management concepts. After heavy rainfalls up to the physically possible (406 liters /m² /d) a number of general hospitals in the Dresden region were flash-flooded at 8/12 and 13/2002 and 100 patients were transferred to the safe classified UHD, among them 20 critically ill. While the waters still raised, by decision of the incident command 1,200 patients from the UHD were evacuated one day later.

Starting August 16 the "empty" **UHD supplied shuttle teams to perform specialized care** in safe general hospitals as well as in auxiliary hospitals, set up on the safe periphery of the flooded area. Furthermore **teams were established by UHD for additional ground and airborne EMS support** in cooperation with the districts in need and the armed forces. Unlike in previous events it appeared that road accidents failed to happen so that, the hospital's reduced in-care capacities turned out to be less of a problem than expected. But it was the **flooding of roads (and the closure of bridges)** that posed a particular challenge for the evacuation and shuttle teams.

Lessons already been learned in leadership, shared mental models, hospital networks, and quality management by the time of disaster onset beyond medical skills turned out to be extremely valuable to all concerned parties. The authors of chapter 11 were part of the operations command within the UHD and do not only describe the events between August 11 and August 20, 2002 as a kind of a captains log, but also shed light on the organizational backgrounds. Just like logistic structures are challenged in such an extreme situation, professional and personal relations are tested. Those who were a part of it got to know each other better.

This chapter completes the overview on the Dresden team management activities, exemplifying the trans regional responsibilities of a university hospital. Business excellence models such as the **EFQM- Model**, likewise, claim for companies´ **business results in favor of the society** [2], which in this sense are met by the UHD and will even be considerably extended by implementing "Carus consilium Sachsen".

CONCLUSION

In the Dresden way of thinking **team management is one key success factor for hospitals in the future**. We have the unique situation of a university hospital that besides its core competencies of excellent patient treatment, also focuses on team- and quality management within a **up to date understanding of employees roles, characterized by meaning and leeway being managed by individuals with emotional intelligence**.

The commitment of the hospital management board to team oriented leadership in a high risk organization is demonstrated by the institution of a second leadership circle (Führungskreis II/ FK II). This leadership circle consists of senior physicians of all departments, who on one side face the true daily problems beyond politics, independently from the board of department chairmen, but on the other side are particularly trained in business administration issues. This book presents ambitious team- oriented and solutions which in parts are the result of FK II projects. Besides the **theoretically sound considerations**, projects and **practice proven concepts** are presented by specialists in their fields.

REFERENCES

[1]   Bleicher K. Future perspectives of organizational development. ZfO 1990;(3):152.

[2]   European Foundation for Quality Management. Introduce Excellence. Brüssel: EFQM; 2003.

[3]   Albrecht DM, Töpfer A. Erfolgreiches Changemanagement im Krankenhaus. 1 ed. Heidelberg: Springer; 2006.

[4]   Kaplan R, Norton D. The Balanced Scorecard. Translating Strategy Into Action. 1 ed. Boston: Harvard Business School Press; 1996.

[5]   Hilb M. Integriertes Personalmanagement. 14 ed. München: Luchterhand; 2005.

[6]   Goleman D. Emotional Intelligence. New York: Bentam Books; 1995.

[7]   Drucker PF. The Practice of Management. New York: Harper & Row; 1954.

[8]   Luft J, Ingham H. The Johari Window, a graphic model for interpersonal relations. Los Angeles: University of California; 1955.

[9]   Van den Bossche P. Minds in teams. Maastricht: Datawyse; 2006.

[10]   Muller M, Bergmann B, Koch T, Heller A. [Dynamic decision making in emergency medicine. Example of paraplegia after a traffic accident]. Anaesthesist 2005 Aug;54(8):781-6.

[11]   Dissmann PD, Le CS. The experience of Teesside helicopter emergency services: doctors do not prolong prehospital on-scene times. Emerg Med J 2007 Jan;24(1):59-62.

[12]   Miller GA. The magic number seven plus / minus two. Psychol Rev 1956;63:81-2.

[13]   Deming WE. Out of the Crisis. New York: McGraw-Hill; 1986.

[14]   Töpfer A. Six Sigma. 3 ed. Berlin: Springer; 2004.

[15]   Kopetsch T. Trek of physicians: Attractions from abroad. Dtsch Arztebl 2008;105(14):716-8.

[16]   Schwab S, Vatankhah B, Kukla C, Hauchwitz M, Bogdahn U, Furst A, et al. Long-term outcome after thrombolysis in telemedical stroke care. Neurology 2007 Aug 28;69(9):898-903.

[17]   Lavery G. Effective Disaster Communication. In: Farmer JC, Jimenez EJ, Talmor DS, Zimmerman JL, editors. Fundamentals in Disaster Management.Des Plaines/ IL: Society of Critical Care Medicine; 2003. p. 9-20.

[18]   Rochlin GI, La Porte T.R., Roberts K.H. The Self-Designing High-Reliability Organization- Aircraft Carrier Flight Operations at Sea. Naval War College Review 1998;51(3).

[19]   Chandler A. Strategy and Structure: Chapters in the history of industrial enterprise. New York: Doubleday; 1962.

ISBN 978-1-60692-307-8

Chapter 2

TEAM MANAGEMENT AS FUTURE KEY FACTOR OF SUCCESS IN HOSPITALS – THE CEO′S VIEW

Detlev-Michael Albrecht

CEO University Hospital Carl Gustav Carus
University of Technology, Dresden, Germany

ABSTRACT

At present, utilizing advanced economic and staff leadership know how must be concern of all process participants in the hospital besides excellent medical task management. The earlier the organization is penetrated by a spirit of service, quality and patient satisfaction the higher is the competitive advantage. Problems in the penetration of the organization with strategic goals can be opposed by means of transparent communication, in both directions top-down and bottom-up.

The key success factor is level of the middle management [1] whose work must first be aligned to the strategic goals of the hospital and second must be phased which each other. This may be achieved by timed objective agreements and respective incentives. Further, in particular in the hospital with its diverse structures and tasks a second leadership circle of the middle management is an invaluable tool to facilitate communication and to generate sustained competitive advantages by close strategy driven process oriented organization.

STRATEGY WITHIN THE FRAMEWORK OF THE NEW G-DRG REIMBURSEMENT SYSTEM

Until recently German hospitals were far away from economic practice, because reimbursement was based upon length of hospital stay and, thus, erroneous incentives dominated patient and case management. The aim of modernizing German health care system in 2003 was to keep the level of quality or even improve it, and at the same time reduce total national health care expenses. This goal in particular was set for the sector of hospital care which makes one third of total annually expenses of the public healthcare assurance system.

To achieve these goals new concepts which have proven their value in other fields of professional business had and have to be implemented into public hospital health care. In contrast to evolution of professional business the development of health care management has to be achieved in fast motion. The future will reveal if developmental mistakes can be avoided by learning from history of economy [2-7] or if we have to bow into particular inevitable errors. Regarding the flawed professional management in the majority of hospitals it can be taken for granted that without a culture of learning from the best and seeking for the feasible, which is standard in other professions, enormous resources will be wasted.

In view of staff development and team leadership, besides excellence in medical care and nursing, economic understanding has inevitably to be put into practice. The key factor that will keep one hospital at the market is optimization of process quality and its resource utilization. Hence, the current competition situation between hospitals, when earnings for the same procedure are fixed at one average level, can be described as a competition for best resource utilization. However, inflating economic, management, and controlling departments in healthcare institutions is misleading. Rather, economic understanding of all process contributors and sustained strategy driven structures [2;3;6] and acting will determine long term success. The earlier one healthcare unit transforms into a strategy driven process oriented organization the sustained is the competitive advantage.

Thinking in categories of competition, desiring for a clear strategy, handy concepts of implementation and, most important, rapid and sustained realization was unknown to the majority of German hospitals.

In this regard two questions require clarification:

- Is the management of a traditional hospital able to perform professional leadership, to overcome newly occurring problems and challenges?
- Will the management of the hospital be rapidly able to initiate the broad changes which were found to be necessary under motivation and inclusion of all important stakeholders, aiming to achieve the desired change with a minimum of avoidable frictions and frustrations?

The first question can clearly be answered in that regard that professional management structures in most hospitals are flawed. The main cause for this is the already mentioned historic development in hospital leadership without higher requirements or challenges, and, thus, low pressure to gain business excellence. Further, medical and nursing management representing two of three groups of hospital top management had no gained knowledge or experience in economics so far and mainly were interested in a professional driven lobby. The third part of hospital top management represented by the head of administration department and responsible for "economics" was mainly concerned with accounting, investing and costing. Thus, competition oriented strategic management so long was never the focus of German hospital top management. The mentioned administrative activities are nonetheless important for healthcare organizations; however, due to their retrospective nature they do not suffice for coping future challenges. The second question seamlessly fits to that idea. Key feature of professional management is early recognition of forthcoming developments and risks and response by well aimed change management, instead of negating threatening evolutions and falling into a state of paralysis.

During the present phase of change in health care politics, persons or organizations in charge of hospitals in Germany should be advised to scrutinize their strategic positioning – in the case it has been defined consciously at all. Moreover, in first line the internal resources which have not yet been employed have to be analyzed and work force which until now is not recognized within the organizational structure shall be utilized. Hospitals hesitating in which direction and with which velocity the new system will develop will be among the losers. The dam is broken; now it is the major goal forward thinking to rate scenarios and to set into action internal change mechanisms. Internal organizational restructuring, tailored therapies meeting the patients´ demands, switching from thinking in department structures to a workflow along clinical pathways as well as much stronger service and customer orientation will be key factors. Figure 1 shows 15 steps to successful hospital management [8].

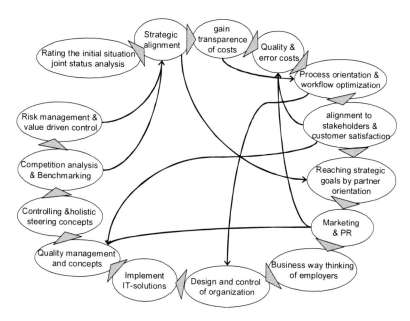

Figure 1. 15 step checklist to improve hospital management (adopted from [8]).

In this regard the emotional discussion, weather patients are customers is misleading. Patients have at least to be handled as customers, because their claims for service, adherence to schedules, and quality are those of customers. Further, in non emergency cases patients show the same mobility and have acquired a high level of medical knowledge about their illness and the hospital. Thus, even within the public healthcare insurance, patients as customers desire for best value for their insurance dues.

STRUCTURE FOLLOWS PROCESS FOLLOWS STRATEGY

The fifth main prerequisite for victory:
"The win will go to the one, whose soldiers share the same conviction."

Sunzi 500 A.D. [9]

The politically favored economic primacy in the health care system has lead to increased competition for patients among service providers and the goal of designing patient friendly processes that are timely, uninterrupted, service-oriented, quality assured, and provided with an efficient use of personnel and resources [8;10]. The required efficiency increase can only be achieved by optimizing medical, as well as non-medical sub-processes of inpatient treatment, with simultaneously higher quality and patient satisfaction in terms of an outperformance [11;12].

Such an approach can only work if the organization establishes a common goal in the form of a vision and strategy, if the goal is broadly communicated to employees on all levels and if the employees accept [13] and live it [10]. Since it cannot be taken for granted that service providers are intrinsically motivated to comply with a specific strategy without any self-interest [14], a performance-related compensation is viewed as a critical success factor of the health care system. [10]

German hospitals with their standard pay schedules do not practice a culture of objective oriented leadership or management by objectives. Some clinics, such as the University Hospital Dresden, changed their legal form prior to the introduction of DRG in order to be able to offer their employees contracts outside the negotiated standard pay schedules and to make parts of the annual salary contingent upon performance.

Already in the 1960s, Chandler [3] described an organizational principle in which the organization's structure must continuously be aligned with its value adding process. This process, as a result of operative management, must also always be aligned with the strategic management goals.

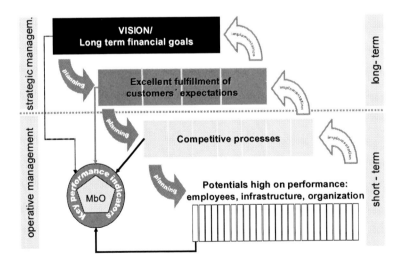

Figure 2. Alignment of individual objectives with the organizational strategy: Top- down planning phase, bottom up implementing phase (MbO = management by objectives).

The organization's top priority is to guarantee its sustained existence in the marketplace. External opportunities and risks (e.g., market position, customer value) must be recognized by strategic management, balanced with the organization's strengths and weaknesses (processes, profitability) [8], and, thus, identified as future success or risk potentials [15].

Operative process planning and organizational development are aligned within the context of the strategic planning process (Figure 2). Once these processes have been clearly defined, it is possible to develop an organizational structure that is completely aligned with these processes [3].

The implementation of the corporate concept works the other way around, since the process performance is based on the existing structure and workforce, and uses corresponding incentive and even punitive systems. Throughout the year, the operative controlling department checks if the objectives of the operative plans are reached and if the resources are used appropriately. On a higher level, strategic controlling verifies if the strategies are feasible and can be implemented. As a last step, if the preceding controlling entities did not provide sufficient counterbalance, the objective might have to be revised.

Within the context of management by objectives (MbO), described by Drucker as early as the 1950s as "*one of the most important jobs of effective management*" [2;16], this means that systems involving agreements on objectives and incentives can only benefit the organization, if they are aligned with the corporate vision and strategy. Business excellence models such as the EFQM operationalize this point of view and expand MbO with the aspects of innovation and learning [17].

Systems based on management by objectives and performance measurements were introduced in many organizations in the 1990s [18] in order to close the gap between strategic and operative management. The problems surrounding the implementation of the corporate strategy into the operative day-to-day business are compensated here through the interface of individual agreements on objectives. The Ernst & Young study "Health Care 2020" considers the introduction of such performance based compensation systems as critical success factor for strategic hospital management [10].

Steering the work force of the middle and upper management of a hospital (chief physicians, senior physicians, chief residents) through management by objectives has, aside from the already mentioned advantage of linking strategic and operative management, the advantage that strategic objectives are, basically in the bottom-up system, quantified into a few task-appropriate key figures, making it possible to verify achieved objectives with respect to a specific assignment. The deciding factor is, however, that strategies are broken down across hierarchies and the responsibility for the results of a sub-area of the strategy can be assigned to an individual employee (fig.2).

Problems [1]:
- **Vision barrier;** only 5% of the employees understand the corporate strategy.
- **Human barrier;** only 25% of the managers are offered incentives relating to the implementation of the strategy
- **Resource barrier;** 60% of organizations do not link their budget to the strategy
- **Management barrier;** 85% of the top managers take less than one hour per month to discuss strategy.

Kaplan and Norton address the problems relating to employee acceptance of the corporate vision and present a correspondingly robust formulation and controlling instrument for objectives in the form of the balance scorecard (BSC) [1]. To deal with these problems, the BSC applies the strategy to the individual employee by introducing an operational, multi-dimensional ratio system. Accordingly, this instrument necessitates the development of a strategy.

Aside from leading to an optimization of the process, the BSC focuses on the value drivers in the business units responsible for the results, and requires and supports a standardized and meaningful internal reporting system for the overall organization that is aligned with the strategy. Regarding the use of the BSC for the management of surgeries, Schüpfer is suggesting the indicators presented in Table 1.

Table 1. Process controlling through early and late indicators in accordance with BSC (source [19])

	BSC Suggestion			
	Innovation	Process	Customer	Finances
Early Indicator	Error Management	Standardized Processes	Close Contact with Referring Physicians	Capacity Utilization
Late Indicator	Number of Liability Cases	Wait Times for Surgeries	Patient Satisfaction	Annual Performance

Regarding the question what the top- management would do otherwise in change processes when they could decide again a study of M+M Management and Marketing in US excellence companies found, according to the findings of Kaplan and Norton, that they would much more intensively care for the middle management [8].

It was always supposed that the middle management would understand the background for change processes and would advocate and support it. This was not the case. The necessity, however, was recognized and ensured too late. Main obstacles in change processes are not time pressure, merely optimizing of sub-processes, leadership or communicative behavior, rather it was blockage by the middle management. One may suppose that in hospitals the same situation will prevail. Because only a low fluctuation of staff is present (except residents or other in-training personnel) successful change processes must refer to motivation and integration of all levels of management.

The middle management has the role of a transmission belt between top-management and employees and, likewise, as driver of the change process. To ensure that they actively take that role in favor of the strategy, the top management must prepare them sufficiently and integrate them into the process of analysis, construction, and change, as depicted in Figure 1.

Within the change process interchange of experience and shoulder to shoulder stance within the middle management is of importance. The latter can effectively be reached when the middle management is not longer an amorphous mass but when they are affiliated as members of a second leadership circle as new organizational unit of hospital management. Reaching commitment for change processes in the middle management is, thus, the main goal of the second leadership circle. However, it must be the objective of the top management that this new organizational unit works efficiently in terms of strategy oriented projects beyond being another lame duck discussion club within the organization.

CONCLUSION

In business areas with high change rates and -velocity one policy is well known: "The only constant in our field is change". This policy however is flawed by the fact that under these circumstances employees might have no reason to participate in every wave of change actively, because shortly another change is expected to impend. The emotional effect has to be taken into account and going a flexible "living example" by the top management is one of the main tasks. Thus, change processes are to be well terminated and should be followed by phases of relative stability. This defined alternation between stability and change is at the same time a measure improving the confidence into the competency of the hospital top management.

REFERENCES

[1]   Kaplan R, Norton D. The Balanced Scorecard. Translating Strategy Into Action. 1 ed. Boston: Harvard Business School Press; 1996.
[2]   Drucker PF. The Practice of Management. New York: Harper & Row; 1954.
[3]   Chandler A. Strategy and Structure: Chapters in the history of industrial enterprise. New York: Doubleday; 1962.
[4]   Argyris C, Schön D.A. Organizational Learning II. Theory, Method, and Practice. Boston: Addison-Wesley; 1996.
[5]   Herzberg F. Work and the Nature of Man. Cleveland: World Publishing Co.; 1966.
[6]   Maslow A. Motivation and Personality. New York: Harper & Row; 1954.
[7]   Taylor FW. The Principles of Scientific Management. New YOrk: 1911.
[8]   Albrecht DM, Töpfer A. Erfolgreiches Changemanagement im Krankenhaus. 1 ed. Heidelberg: Springer; 2006.
[9]   Sunzi W. Die Kunst des Krieges. München: Droemer Knaur; 2001.
[10] Böhlke R, Söhnle N, Viering S. Gesundheitsversorgung 2020. Frankfurt: Ernst & Young; 2005.
[11] Sachverständigenrat. Finanzierung und Nutzerorientierung - Gutachten des Sachverständigenrats für die Konzertierte Aktion im Gesundheitswesen. 1 ed. Baden Baden: Nomos- Verlag; 2003.
[12] Siegmund F, Berry M, Martin J, Geldner G, Bauer M, Bender HJ, et al. Entwicklungsstand im OP-Management - Eine Analyse in deutschen Krankenhäusern im Jahr 2005. Anaesthesiologie & Intensivmedizin 2006;47(12):743-50.
[13] Beitz H. Zielvereinbarungen. Das Handbuch für den Vorgesetzten, Loseblattsammlung.Bonn: Fachverlag für Recht und Führung; 2001.
[14] Hobbes T. Leviathan. London: 1651.
[15] Gälweiler A, Schwaninger M. Strategische Unternehmensführung. 2 ed. Campus Verlag; 2001.
[16] Drucker PF. Das Geheimnis effizienter Führung. Harvard Businesss Manager 2005;(3):7-14.
[17] European Foundation for Quality Management. Excellence einführen. Brüssel: EFQM; 2003.

[18] Brown DM, Laverick S. Measuring Corporate Performance. Long Range Planning 1994;27(4):89-98.

[19] Schüpfer G, Bauer M, Scherzinger B, Schleppers A. Controllinginstrumente fur OP-Manager. Anaesthesist 2005 Aug;54(8):800-7.

ISBN 978-1-60692-307-8
© 2009 Nova Science Publishers, Inc.

Chapter 3

SUPPORT OF MULTITASKING MEDICAL TEAM LEADERSHIP USING PERFORMANCE MEASUREMENT SYSTEMS*

Axel R. Heller[1], Thea Koch[1] and Maria Eberlein-Gonska[2]
[1]Department of Anesthesiology & Critical Care Medicine,
[2]Department of Quality Management, University Hospital Carl Gustav Carus,
University of Technology, Dresden, Germany
*This work is part of a Modular Article by A. Heller within the Healthcare Management studies for MBA- degree at the Dresden International al University, Dresden, Germany

ABSTRACT

One major problem of business management is to **align the workforce of the employees with the strategy** as well as the long term goals of the company top management. Within the German healthcare system such way of business thinking not emerged until the German diagnoses related reimbursement system was introduced in 2003. One would suppose, that the competition between the hospitals for patients would nowadays have set hospitals under such evolution pressure, that **formulating a company vision and strategy is imperative**. The first question persons or organizations in charge of hospitals in Germany should, thus, be asked, if strategic positioning in their hospital has been defined consciously at all.

The level of hierarchy which in particular must be addressed is the **middle management**. This party **decides over success or failure of any strategy driven activity** of the top management by their degree of commitment and involvement. It is therefore indebatable, that hospitals in the same way as successful companies, have to generate a **WIN-WIN condition with their middle management**, namely the Heads of Departments and the level of medical consultants.

Management by objectives (MBO) is the key link between the companies' strategy, individual assignments, and performance. Kaplan and Norton in 1996 introduced the balanced scorecard (BSC) as a means to overcome the deficits of strategic alignment of the middle management, to automate MBO and bring it down to the individual employee. Introduction of BSC in most cases, however, demands implementation within the whole company to enable maximum utility.

This chapter besides general backgrounds on MBO discusses efforts and utility of performance measurement systems and finally provides a BSC- like management chart to align activities of the middle management to the departments goals.

MANAGEMENT BY OBJECTIVES IN THE HEALTH CARE SYSTEM

Objectives are anticipated results
F. Malik [1]

Due to the implementation of the DRG system for inpatient care, the increasing number of outpatient procedures, and the resulting reduction of financial margins, medical inpatient care must be made more efficient [2;3]. The new organizational concepts have especially changed the scope and areas of **shared responsibility** for anesthesiologists, whose focus for quite some time had been limited to the immediate peri-operative period, in the direction of a **comprehensive treatment philosophy in cooperation with their surgical partners** [4], ranging from acute pain therapy [5] to fast track dietary [6] and rehabilitation concepts. Therefore, this kind of strategy-compliant cutting-edge performance must be also be included in their performance evaluation, in addition to the standard performance parameter for anesthesiologists (number of cases/anesthesia minutes).

Since it cannot be taken for granted that service providers are intrinsically motivated to comply with a specific strategy without any self-interest [7], a **performance-related compensation is viewed as a critical success factor of the health care system**. [3] German hospitals with their standard pay schedules do not practice a culture of management by objectives. Some clinics, such as the University hospital of Dresden, however, changed their legal form [8] prior to the introduction of DRG. Besides other advantages the legal form of a *Corporation of public law* enables to offer the employees contracts outside the negotiated standard pay schedules and to make parts of the annual salary contingent upon performance.

The starting point for this article was the need for the development of an allocation formula for the inclusion of senior staff members at the clinic for anesthesiology and intensive care at the UHD (Dresden University Hospital) into the private liquidation pool of the Head of Department. Up until that point, the pool's funds had been allocated at the director's discretion.

MANAGEMENT BY OBJECTIVES – SYSTEMS IN PRACTICE

"There are only a few factors that distinguish competent management from incompetent management, such as the ability to weigh objectives against each other"
P. Drucker [9]

The theoretical and practical background expressed by Chandler's quotation **"structure follows process follows strategy"** [10] has been thoroughly discussed from the CEO's view in chapter 2 and the necessity to do so is as old as competition exists *(Sunzi 500 A.D) [11]*. As early as in the 1960s, Chandler deduced that the organization's structure has continuously to support its value adding process, rather than the other way round, which is regularly sad reality. And, second, the process must be constructed to serve the strategies demands which itself is driven by the idea of prosperous sustained existence in the marketplace. Thus, **alignment of the employees workforce with the strategy** as well as the long term goals of the company top management e.g., by Management by Objectives (MbO) is *"one of the most important jobs of effective management"* [9;12] (P. Drucker). Managemend systems such as the balanced scorecard (BSC) [13] or business excellence models such as EFQM operationalize this point of view implementing various key performance indicators (see chapter 2; Figure 2) and expand MbO with the aspects of innovation and learning [14].

There are several factors that need to be taken into consideration when implementing MbO systems [15]. Since the goal of the MbO system is to implement the strategic corporate objectives as well as the objectives of the employees at the same time, the objectives for each organizational unit and each employee are determined in conjunction with them. These objectives should be "SMART" (specific, measurable, achievable, relevant, and timed) [9;16]:

S - Specific (to the respective department)
M - Measurable (clear parameters)
A - Achievable (attainable)
R - Relevant (workable)
T - Timed (clear time limit)

Key properties of agreement on objectives

The Corporate Objectives are Expressed as the Sum of the Individual Objectives of All Employees

The Quality Management business unit of the UHD then structures the employees' objectives in accordance with Figure 1. Employees must provide their individual objectives for the five listed dimensions and coordinate these with the manager of the respective business unit, who then also includes objectives from a corporate strategy perspective. At the end of the agreed period [17], there will be a dialogue about the extent to which the objectives have been achieved.

Aside from offering the ability to assign clear objectives to individual employees, MbO is a particularly useful way to increase motivation within the business unit, if it is linked to material or immaterial incentives. In addition, achieved objectives and successes are the best motivation for agreeing to additional tasks and for further development [1]. This holds true both for the individual level, as well as the team and corporate level. It is therefore suggested to word the final objective in the perfect tense.

Example:

- *Objective: The business process Parts-Sales is optimized within the context of the "sunflower" project. The interfaces between departments 47, 48, 50, and 51 are thereby redefined, designed in an organizational manner, and clearly regulated.*

- *Benchmark: The current throughput time of 12 minutes is decreased to 8 minutes. (<7 minutes: Objective has been exceeded, >9 minutes: Objective has not been achieved).*

At the same time, it is important to make sure that not only the ultimate objectives are defined, but that interim objectives define individual milestones necessary to reach the objective [16].

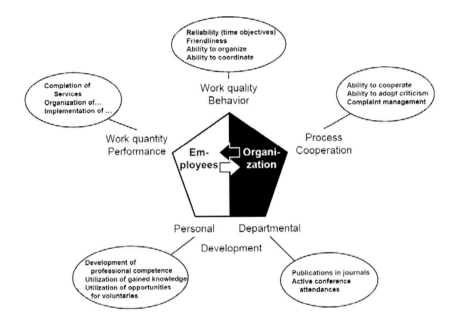

Figure 1. Requirement pentagon for the annual objectives of individual employees including examples (illustration as modified per [15;16]).

Aside from the criteria of "yes/no" and quantitative criteria, it is also customary to use three-step (traffic light), five-step (academic grades) or percentage scales. In contrast to the categorical evaluation of "objective met/not met", scales allow for a graduated evaluation and incentive structure, so that also *almost* reached objectives can, likewise, be honored.

In the past, some of the main problems with agreements on objectives were that they did not focus on real objectives, but activities, leading to a confusion with operational planning, or that the objectives were dictated instead of mutually agreed upon. In addition, it is possible to agree on objectives with employees without having a defined corporate strategy, but these are then not stringently linked to corporate success, and are "objectless" in this respect.

Some problems are also caused by the lack of horizontal alignment of the objectives across the departments or employees, since priorities, resources, and processes are then not aligned and the MbO potential for the organization is not fully utilized. In addition, MbO loses its meaning if there is no discussion about which objectives have been achieved, or if there is no incentive system.

On the other hand, it is important to make sure that the objectives satisfy important employee needs (material/immaterial), that the achievement of the objective is (only) related to *individual* performance, and that the required performance can really be achieved through individual effort. The equitable distribution should also take this into consideration (Figure 2). [18]

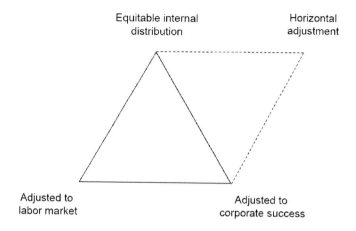

Figure 2. "Magic" equitable distribution double triangle (modified per [18])

Experience gained during the past five years with the MbO and performance-related compensation systems have shown that objectives were not designed in a multi-dimensional manner as shown by the BSC or in Figures 1 & 2, and that there was merely a simple project/ or performance relation. These kinds of objectives presuppose that behavior, cooperation, and development-related aspects do not require any changes. Accordingly, the senior staff members that are to conduct the meetings during which the objective agreements are developed should be sufficiently prepared in order to use the MbO tool effectively, and in accordance with the corporate strategy and the internal equitable distribution (Figure 2).

Examples from the years 2003-2007:

- Evaluation of anesthesiological services based on patient satisfaction and side effects, physical indicators, and clinical outcome *Period: 08/01/2003-12/31/2003*
- Participation in the clinic's on-call service *Period: 08/01/2003-2007*
- Development of a continuing education and certification concept for in-house residents in anesthesiology *Period 08/01/2003-05/30/2004*
- Presentation of a clinical research concept, incorporating personnel resources and material costs for 2004/05 *Period: 05/12/2004- 10/31/2004*
- Development of a scanner-readable anesthesia documentation protocol for the collection of revenue-related information with evaluability of scientific questions. Presentation of the protocol including cost calculation and pilot tests *Period: 05/12/2004-11/30/2004*
- Implementation of the developed continuing education concept for physicians at the clinic starting July 2004. Coordination of the continuing education events and documentation of the discussion relating to the test results. *Term: 05/12/2004- 04/30/2005*
- Development of a quality report and an annual report for the clinic 2004/04 *Period: 03/03/2005- 04/30/2005*

- Process optimization in the anesthesia department by evaluating the key figures related to the utilization of operating rooms and application of statistical process control algorithms. *Period: 03/03/2005- 10/30/2005*
- Pandemic influenza preparedness plan for the UHD *Period: 3/2006- 4/2006*
- Profit contribution calculation for anesthesiology services in relation to the DRG matrix for Top 10 DRGs at the UHD. *Period: 3/2006- 4/2007*

RETURNS ON THE INVESTMENT INTO PERFORMANCE MEASUREMENT SYSTEMS

In natural systems, the performance characteristics are usually normally distributed (fig. 4). [19] Therefore, it can be assumed that this also applies to the performance of senior staff members in an organization. Under this premise, 68% of the senior staff members will do average work, while 13.5 or 2.5%, respectively, will do very good or exceptional work. It is to be expected that 16% of the senior staff members will do far below-average work.

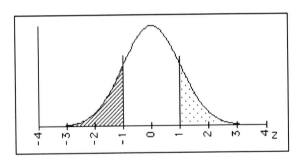

Figure 4. Normal distribution including standard deviation, (y-axis: Number of employees, x-axis: Performance quality): Average employees (white), below-average employees (shaded), above-average employees (dotted). Outstanding employees (positive/negative) outside of the 2 sigma range.

Since an MbO and performance measurement system tells that most of the senior staff members do average work, Malik doubts the usefulness of extremely standardized algorithms, particularly, because the *type* of evaluation, e.g., time-consuming system bureaucracy, replaces the originally intended evaluation *content*. [1] He concedes that a standardized evaluation is acceptable and useful, only in cases where the employee requirement profile is relatively standardized.

Ideally, the incentive amount should correspond to the employee's performance. There is a heated debate, however, about how to measure performance. One of the main aspects of this debate is that an employee's work can only be considered as performance, if it relates to the organization's objectives [1]. This congruency problem between corporate and individual objectives can be solved, however, through the use of clear, strategically driven objectives.

There are many different performance evaluation systems. [1;13;18;20;21] What they all have in common is a more or less administratively elaborate, standardized key figure model (Figure 5), focusing on employee or organizational areas, where weak points are suspected.

Considering the strategic conditions already outlined the categorizing of employees into salary brackets (Figure 5), which are typically used for civil servants, is insufficient, especially regarding the establishment of individually customized performance incentives for the hospitals' senior staff members. Any improvements that resulted from switching from the BAT [German civil service pay scale] to the TVÖD [pay agreement for the German civil service] for hospitals were only a first step in the right direction. It is necessary to use more precise and complex processes, even though they may be costly and time consuming, to adequately quantify the individual labor value and at the same time guarantee an equitable internal distribution (Figure 2). Particularly organizations located in former Eastern German states still having around 10% lower compensation scales related to Western Germany must offset this disadvantage with regard to labor market and personnel recruiting implementing forward-looking incentive systems [3].

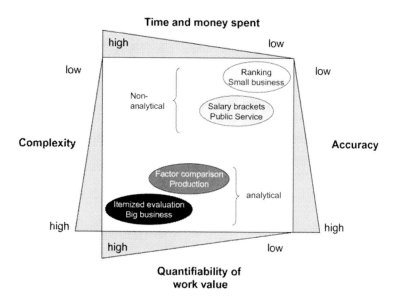

Figure 5. Relationship between time and money spent, accuracy, complexity, and quantification benefits in evaluation systems (modified as per [18]).

The main prerequisite for objective-oriented performance management is the existence of a defined workflow in terms of standard operational procedures (SOP) or clinical treatment pathways. [2;22;23] Current benchmarking data from German hospitals [24] indicate that only 10.1% of all participating hospitals have full-time OR management and OR controlling services. This shows that reattribution of departmental results, absolutely critical for corporate success, is not taking place. As a result, the strategic corporate objectives, if any, cannot be mirrored by the performance data, eliminating the possibility of performance control.

This may lead to a serious problem for the hospital, if it is not able to operate efficiently and if its senior staff members are not willing to perform accordingly. Malik explains that in this event even motivation would not suffice to improve the achievement of objectives. [1] Two considerations seem indicated here: For one, the ability to perform and the willingness to perform are subjective parameters and work performance is not interchangeable with efficiency. By benchmarking with comparable departments, the figures become more objective [25]. But he also fails to consider whether the current level of employee performance is caused by an already existing motivation culture, and if they are mutually dependant. In such cases, a long-term personnel development concept comes into play, which, for example, could be structured in accordance with the personnel/portfolio approach [18]. This approach transfers insights about the product life cycle to the personnel development area by exposing employees for as long as possible and repeatedly to personal growth phases by taking the respective internal rotation measures, characterized by meaning, leeway, and fun.

AGREEMENTS ON OBJECTIVES FOR THE CLINIC FOR ANESTHESIA/ UHD MISSION AND VISION

Vision of the Clinic for Anesthesia and Intensive Care / UHD [26]

- We stand for medical, scientific, and process-related top level service and are a national competency leader in providing perioperative services in anesthesia, intensive care, as well as emergency medical care, and pain therapy in close cooperation with the surgical partners.
- We support scientific progress through our own research, participation in international competence networks and the continuous transfer of knowledge into patient care.
- By offering structured continuing education opportunities we qualify our colleagues for acting with professional competency, aware of their responsibility for their patients, and to work cost-effective.

Mission of the Clinic for Anesthesia [26]

- Excellence in anesthesia and pain therapy care, allowing all kinds of surgeries and diagnostic procedures for patients in our care
- Treatment of seriously ill patients through humane and professional intensive care and on a superior international level
- Conduct innovative, clinically relevant, internationally recognized research and patient-centered teaching
- We are a European center for continuing education of medical specialists and provide our employees with the skills necessary to become top performers in their field
- By acting in a process-oriented manner and actively shaping cross-disciplinary centers, we contribute to the optimization of the treatment results and revenue assurance.

The core task of the clinic for anesthesiology is to guarantee the provision of anesthesia services at the UHD. In addition, it operates an interdisciplinary and cardio-surgical intensive care unit and a day clinic for pain therapy. In 2005 and 2006, approx. 23,000 anesthesia services were rendered per year (3.9 million anesthesia minutes), 23% of which related to regional anesthesia procedures.

The wording of the vision and mission statements makes clear that the position as a university clinic and the respective claim to excellence regarding research, teaching, patient care, and cost-effective operations leads unavoidably to conflicting objectives. This positioning clearly contradicts the mandate that the agreements on objectives should be free from conflicting objectives. [1;16;27] Basically, this problem could be solved if only medical specialists could focus in all areas on research, teaching, *or* patient care. This organizational model does not, however, correspond to the academic thought as formulated by Humboldt 200 years ago that research, teaching, and application depend on each other and feed off each other and that they constitute a strategic advantage for the future. [3]

The clinic for anesthesia at the UHD is convinced, however, that its mission should be seen precisely in the latter mentioned extremely intellectually exciting context because it is keen on developing its employees and executives in this spirit. All employees are offered the opportunity of a 360 degree function throughout their career at the clinic and are challenged to take advantage of it.

Of course, not *all* objectives can be pursued on an equally high level at the same time. Therefore, focus must be set on a specific assignment on an annual basis within the agreement with the individual employee. Since the activities of the lower management level (unit supervisors) in the anesthesia clinic are relatively standardized, it is possible to draft an evaluation matrix expressing strategy-compliant performance in a weighted manner. It seems legitimate to always carry out a 360 degree evaluation, because this allows those strategy-compliant performances that are not explicitly outlined in job descriptions and annual objectives to be honored.

PROCESS

Anesthesia's role within the core process is depicted in Figure 6. Our supportive, value-adding process is a basically facultative part of the two main processes diagnostics and therapy within the business process of a DRG and must be incorporated here in a strategic and workflow-oriented manner.

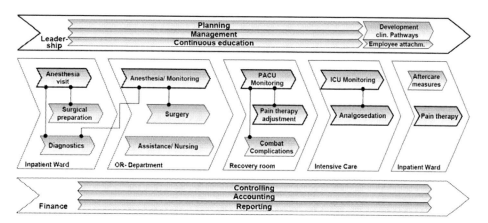

Figure 6. Process landscape of the DRG business process illustrating anesthesia-related work flow from the initial contact to the discharge of the patient.

This chapter goes into quite some detail about patient care in the operating room, because this is where the majority of the full-time physicians 60/72 of the clinic for anesthesia are deployed [28], and because this area is the most cost intensive segment of the business process (also see Figure 11) [29], even though research and teaching as well as intensive care and pain therapy must also be provided by the clinic in accordance with its mission (Figure 7).

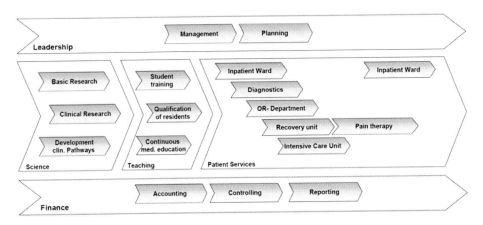

Figure 7. Process landscape illustrating anesthesia's patient services powered by preceding additional academic focuses.

The core process starts with the premedication consultation that takes place one or several days prior to the surgery and ends after the surgery, when the patient is transferred from the operating room. The key figures obtainable from the workflow and useful to operative and strategic management are addressed later on. Due to the many interfaces in the OR area and reciprocal dependencies, there are problems interfering with an orderly and profitable progression on a daily basis. To maximize the usefulness of MbO and process controlling, it is important to identify the respective weak points, monitor them over a certain period of time and address them with the help of organizational measures. Ultimately, the performance of one's own department can only be monitored and managed in terms of benchmarking and its development over time in a strategy-oriented manner.

As already mentioned, only a small number of management-relevant key figures may be included [16;30], which depend on the *individual* performance of the unit supervisor and are not significantly influenced by disturbance variables. Consequently, only very few variables and indicators mentioned in Figure 8 can actually be influenced by a senior staff member of the anesthesiology department. In order to properly structure the process optimization course, it is critical to align the objectives, processes, and priorities of the professional groups and departments involved. This must be done by the senior management. It would seem to make sense to establish an OR-center in terms of a service center in charge of the budget to reduce the interfaces and to address the complex dependencies and problematic areas [31].

In order to gain an integrated overview of the performance of senior staff members in the OR area over a certain period of time, process controlling must be structured in such a way that performance and key figures relating to finances, productivity, process, cost structure, employee and patient satisfaction are readily available; in short, the four dimensions of the Balanced Scorecard [13]. As an alternative to the BSC concept, a business excellence model, e.g., EFQM with its five enabler and four results criteria could also be used [14]. This model differentiates even more between parameters and pays more attention to the interdependency of the various factors.

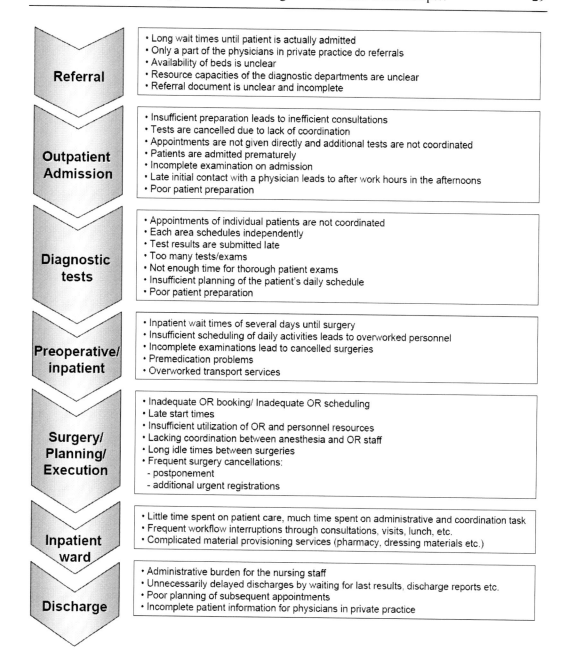

Referral
- Long wait times until patient is actually admitted
- Only a part of the physicians in private practice do referrals
- Availability of beds is unclear
- Resource capacities of the diagnostic departments are unclear
- Referral document is unclear and incomplete

Outpatient Admission
- Insufficient preparation leads to inefficient consultations
- Tests are cancelled due to lack of coordination
- Appointments are not given directly and additional tests are not coordinated
- Patients are admitted prematurely
- Incomplete examination on admission
- Late initial contact with a physician leads to after work hours in the afternoons
- Poor patient preparation

Diagnostic tests
- Appointments of individual patients are not coordinated
- Each area schedules independently
- Test results are submitted late
- Too many tests/exams
- Not enough time for thorough patient exams
- Insufficient planning of the patient's daily schedule
- Poor patient preparation

Preoperative/ inpatient
- Inpatient wait times of several days until surgery
- Insufficient scheduling of daily activities leads to overworked personnel
- Incomplete examinations lead to cancelled surgeries
- Premedication problems
- Overworked transport services

Surgery/ Planning/ Execution
- Inadequate OR booking/ Inadequate OR scheduling
- Late start times
- Insufficient utilization of OR and personnel resources
- Lacking coordination between anesthesia and OR staff
- Long idle times between surgeries
- Frequent surgery cancellations:
  - postponement
  - additional urgent registrations

Inpatient ward
- Little time spent on patient care, much time spent on administrative and coordination task
- Frequent workflow interruptions through consultations, visits, lunch, etc.
- Complicated material provisioning services (pharmacy, dressing materials etc.)

Discharge
- Administrative burden for the nursing staff
- Unnecessarily delayed discharges by waiting for last results, discharge reports etc.
- Poor planning of subsequent appointments
- Incomplete patient information for physicians in private practice

Figure 8. Workflow problems relating to surgery inpatient workflow.

STRUCTURE

After having described the concrete objectives and processes, this section addresses the infrastructure requirements at the UHD and presents the organizational details and job descriptions for senior staff members involved, which were derived from the objectives and

Job Description of the anesthesia unit supervisor

The anesthesia unit supervisor represents the Clinic Director in his respective area of responsibility. Based on his professional and organizational competencies demonstrated to date, the unit supervisor is charged with the management of the unit on a time limited basis. He reports to the Clinic Director, the Chief Medical Director, and the ANE Coordinator with regard to all professional and organizational matters. Unless otherwise agreed upon with the Clinic Director, the unit supervisor provides anesthesiology services for patients with private insurance.

The anesthesia unit supervisor is assigned personnel by the medical director in charge of personnel through the weekly schedule and, if necessary, by the OR Coordinator through his daily disposition. In order to comply with long-ranging educational schedules, it is important to make sure personnel fluctuations are kept to a minimum. If required by the anesthesiological personnel situation and upon consultation with the unit supervisor, the ANE coordinator may requisition staff from the sub department. In this event, it must be assured that the ongoing anesthesias can be completed safely. At the end of the scheduled day, the unit supervisor must verify that all premedications for his area were completed in consultation with the premedication outpatient center.

Tasks / Competencies / Areas of Responsibility

Planning and decision-making responsibility for the execution and efficiency of the daily anesthesia procedures and the OR schedule for his area, taking into consideration the OR status of the UKD and the corporate strategy.

- Up-to-date OR scheduling
  - Realistic OR scheduling / OR utilization
  - Observance of the time periods necessary to prepare the OR for another patient under consideration of technical key figures
  - Additional surgeries/ emergencies in consultation with anesthesiological support staff and the ANE Coordinator
  - Feedback to the ANE Coordinator about the schedule status by 3:00 pm
- Near-term OR scheduling (following work day)
  - Realistic OR capacities for surgeons
  - Reliable working conditions for the employees of the department (working hours, breaks, overtime, advanced training)
  - Adherence to patient appointments and time frames
  - Minimization of non-value-adding activities.
- Quality Assurance
- Continuous improvement process / corporate suggestion system
- Authority to issue directives to employees of the anesthesia department when executing medical/operational processes / compliance with regulations
- Close coordination with all parties involved, anesthesiological support staff, surgical support staff, surgeons, outpatient anesthesia, ANE Coordinator
- Personnel development and advanced training, development and implementation of qualification measures, e.g. development of competency standards, SOPs, patient pathways, monitoring of quality standards
  - Rotation, introductory and exit interviews throughout the year
  - Employee evaluations, to be submitted by 06/30 or 12/31 of every year
- Monitoring and documentation of services and service standards
  - Anesthesia protocols for the department by the end of each month
  - First patient in induction at 7:30 AM
  - Anesthesia surgery- ready (Goal: 08:00 AM)
  - First incision 15 min after surgery ready anesthesia or after 50% of the agreed upon time between surgeries (e.g. between 8:15 AM and 8:25 AM)
  - Agreed versus actual time between surgeries within the department
  - Last suture time of each day and number and total of exceeded times (goal: 3:15 PM), excluding planned late shift ORs

Figure 9. Job description of anesthesia unit supervisor. ANE = Anesthesia dept; UKD = University hospital of Dresden; OR= operation room; SOP= standard operational procedure.

processes. One of the organizational problems the UHD must deal with on a daily basis is its pavilion architecture, a result of the 1901 planning date. Future-oriented constructions, as exemplified by the Greiz hospital, are workflow oriented and *"embed the process into the architecture"* [2]. Due to the structural conditions, the UHD clinic for anesthesia spans over 19 functional areas and involves 49 workstations. The dispersed locations of the surgical and diagnostic areas requiring anesthesia services on the UHD-campus lead to a fragmentation of the work force, long distances, and wait times which is hardly economic. In contrast to a modern surgical center, as was realized for 6 functional areas with 16 operating rooms in building 58/59 of the UHD, the overall personnel dispositions needed to assure patient care as per Section 70 SGB V [Social Security Code V] are disproportionately high.

Usually, for each OR with two to five work stations, one supervisory anesthesiologist must be scheduled in addition to the normal staff including one resident anesthesiologist in each OR. To compensate for shortness of personnel during daily work the anesthesiological coordinator is in charge of an overriding, needs-oriented redistribution of personnel resources to optimize personnel utilization.

MANAGEMENT BY OBJECTIVE TIED TO KEY FIGURES

How should we be organized...
... so that the work the customer is paying us for
is the center of attention and also remains as such?
... so that the work we pay our employees for
can actually be accomplished?
... so that the work top management is being paid for
can actually be accomplished?

F. Malik [1]

With regard to rewarding strategy-compliant behavior of employees, it is of utmost importance that the performance evaluation system is objective. As illustrated by the Johari model (Figure 10), there are inevitably informational asymmetries between the employee and the employer that could lead to conflict and decreased motivation. The employer may be deceived by an average senior staff member, who presents a facade or an image relating to an area to be evaluated (cocky attitude, status symbols, emphasizing his exceptional skills, etc.) [32] in order to get a favorable evaluation and to satisfy his own narcissism [33], even though he is aware of his personal weaknesses.

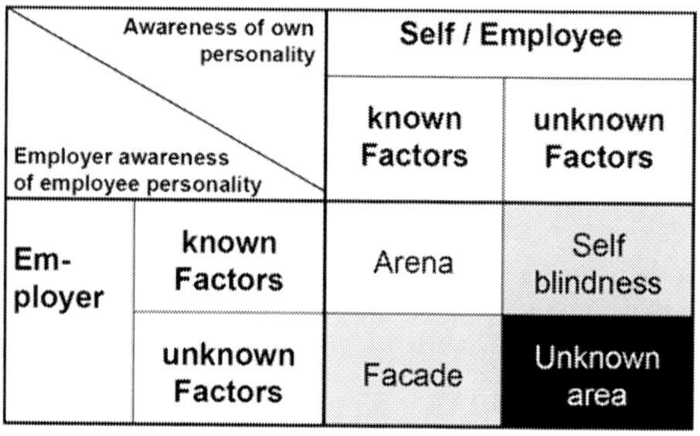

Awareness of own personality / Employer awareness of employee personality		Self / Employee	
		known Factors	unknown Factors
Em-ployer	known Factors	Arena	Self blindness
	unknown Factors	Facade	Unknown area

Figure 10. Johari Model of self evaluation and evaluation by others [34]

If the employee is also unaware of his actual weaknesses, the conflict potential of the evaluation increases. The culture of the organization is particularly affected, if the personal facade/hidden areas are communicated to young employees, often also at the expense of other senior staff members [26]. Therefore, it is absolutely necessary to use - as even possible - an incorruptible, retraceable, and relevant key figure system that can resist hidden and blind areas.

But the organization's objective is *not* control. The question to be asked when implementing performance parameters is not: *"Which areas can we control?"*, but should be: *"What must be controlled so that we can be sufficiently confident that nothing goes seriously wrong?"* [1] In addition, a senior staff member has only a defined span of control, which does not allow for the control of any more complex systems. Miller comes to the conclusion that 7 ± 2 parameters/ tasks can be mastered simultaneously. Any larger number of parameters can only be handled in a sequential manner. [30] Each monitored unit must be restricted to the smallest possible number of benchmarks, since on the one hand control translates into additional work that does not add any value, and on the other hand, depending on its effect on the corporate culture, the employee's confidence and trust might be affected. When selecting relevant parameters, the focus might be the qualitative characteristics of the senior staff member. Correspondingly, Critical to Quality (CTQ) characteristics [35] for the respective senior staff member should be drafted in accordance with the corporate strategy. CTQ should not only be viewed in terms of patient orientation but also to the internal customers (*see Chapter 8*). The decision as to which characteristics are CTQ depends on the corporate strategy, since the employer as customer purchases work performance from the senior staff member. In the end, of course, the corporate strategy must be based on a Voice of the Customer (VOC)- CTQ analysis relating to the patient [14;35].

For the purpose of gathering process data the clinic information system ORBIS (AGFA Healthcare, Munich, Germany) and routine database subsystems [36] provide a sufficient factual background for the evaluation of the unit supervisor.

AVAILABILITY OF HARD AND SOFT KEY FIGURES

Key figures which enable effective process controlling in the OR area are summarized in Table 1. [37] The main controlling premise is that insufficient internal coordination becomes increasingly important, as it leads to increased cost without creating a productive equivalent (idle efforts). Accordingly, the key figures are ranked in accordance with VOC-CTQs having a significant influence on the corporate strategy. [21;35] The performance and key figures, which are to be collected on a regular basis, should, thus, not only be forwarded to the hospital operator as part of the general reporting schedule, but should, as already explained, reflect the strategic achievement of interim objectives.

The corresponding parameters from the perioperative area are adherence to admission and diagnostic schedules, delayed start of surgery, and postponement of procedures that can be scheduled. It is important to **link the collected key figures to horizontally aligned stakeholder agreements on objectives**.

Table 1. Internal summary of process- relevant controlling parameters in the OR management

Objectives of process controlling	Controlling time periods	
	Daily	**Weekly/monthly/annually**
Key figures	Surgical time of attendance Anesth. time of attendance	Surgical time of attendance [A] Anesth. time of attendance [A]
OR utilization	Current OR utilization OR time per room • Core working hrs. • Emergency schedule	Number of surgeries per ORs[1] OR time per room[2] [A] Capacity utilization by • clinic • OR
Resource optimization	Actual time / scheduled time • Anesthesia time • OR time • Employee factor	Personnel utilization [C] • anesthesia time per employee • OR time per employee • time between surgeries per employee Personnel cost per OR time[3] by clinic and professional group [B]
Organizational workflow	First incision time per day Additional surgeries planned per • surgeon • shift ASA corrected ANT per IST [B] • employees • clinic Reasons for delay [B]	Preoperative presence for routine surgeries[4] [A] First incision times by • clinic [A] • surgeon [C] Additional emergency surgeries per [C] • surgeon • shift Surgery cancellations per • clinic [B] • surgeon
Profitability	Incidents (AO) per • clinic • surgeon • anesthesiologist	Case mix per • operating room • surgeon • anesthesiologist
Effectiveness	Time between surgeries per clinic Time between surgeries per physician • surgeon • anesthesiologist ANT per IST[5] by specialty [B]	OR times per clinic (physician); OR times per physician (top 10 procedures) Utilization of the emergency ORs in reference to the time of day IST per InEK IST [B] ANT per InEK ANT [B]
Profitability		Profit contribution by clinic per • operating room • operating hour DRG proceeds/ treatment day/ ANT [B] DRG- proceeds/ treatment day/ IST [B]

ANT = Anesthesia time, IST = Incision-suture time = OR time; SIT = Suture - Incision time = time between surgeries; InEK Institute for the compensation system in hospitals → inferable profitable times from the DRG browser; case mix = sum of case weights; AO = anesthesia observation

[A]   Imperative parameter (operative controlling)
[B]   Sensible parameter (strategic controlling)
[C]   Indicative parameter regarding process optimization

---

[1] Target > 800-1000 p.a. [2]Target >75,000 min p.a. [3]Target < 7.16€ [4]Target < 0.7 days [5]Target< 1.40 ratio [38]

A critical key figure, relevant for the majority of the stakeholders in the OR area, is the normal first incision time. In merely 10% of the operating rooms, surgery starts around 8:00 AM, as mandated by the operating room regulations. Full capacity is gained not before 9:00 AM. The resulting annual monetary losses incurred in this manner in 80-90% of all operating rooms at the expense of the UHD amount to approx. EUR 284,000. Consequently, it should be in the strategic interest of the organization to structure working hour models and agreements on objectives, horizontally aligned between professional groups and clinic, in such a manner that it is possible to start the first surgery of the day around 8:00 AM. Due to the multitude of interfaces, the organization of the OR area as a service center would clearly facilitate these kinds of organizational matters. [31]

STRATEGY-COMPLIANT BEHAVIOR AND BEHAVIOR TO BE LINKED TO INCENTIVES

> *The general who attacks without setting his sights on glory, and who withdraws without being afraid of disgrace, who is only interested in protecting his country and in serving his lord - this general is the gem of the kingdom.*   Sunzi 500 A.D. [11]

In response to the competitive health care market [2;3], the internal treatment pathways of a hospital must be developed in an interprofessional and cross-departmental manner in order to guarantee a smooth workflow (also refer to Figure 8). [39] Since the outpacing strategy (maximized quality with simultaneous cost minimization [21]) is the particularly decisive factor for success in the health care market [2;3], all professional groups, including anesthesia and ancillary staff must be involved in the clinical pathways and their implementation. In this context, corresponding incentive systems are a must [3].

For hospital and departmental innovations, the number of (implemented) improvement suggestions, e.g., the introduction of a postoperative pain concept and implemented standards could be used, since they are CTQ. [35] From a process perspective, the time between the decision and the implementation, as well as the employee compliance (%) with regard to the standard are decisive and could, thus, be appropriate parameters for agreements on objectives. Especially at university clinics, some of the indicators for innovative work include the number of introduced new methods including cost, benefit, and risk evaluations, the number and quality of publications (impact factor), patents, presentations, third party funds and the qualification for additional medical functions. The clinical leadership must pay particular attention to a balanced evaluation of the various items of the 360 degree approach, the measurability of which differs considerably from each other [26].

Since more than half of the medical staff at the clinic is in the process of obtaining their specialist certification and the clinic's vision reflects its clear commitment to advanced training, the performance measurement system should include if and to what extent employees are satisfied with the unit supervisor in its capacity as trainer/mentor. In this context, questions relating to personal work situations of the employees, cooperation and communication with the senior staff member, and his leadership style are of particular interest [2]. In addition, the personal, professional, social, and leadership competencies of persons in leadership positions should be evaluated [18]. For this reason, semi-annual, bilateral evaluations are done for the training supervisor as well as the employees. We have published the questionnaires in book-form as part of a advanced training curriculum for anesthesiologists [40] which has been provided to all employees. Individual meetings to be held at the end of each rotation period between the unit supervisor and the employees and based on the evaluation questionnaires offer a schematized, and therefore objectified and transparent platform to discuss strengths and weaknesses on both sides. The resulting evaluation of the supervisors is included in their performance evaluation.

ABILITY OF KEY FIGURES TO SHOW STRATEGY-COMPLIANT BEHAVIOR - HARD KEY FIGURES

Special regional anesthesia techniques (thoracic epidural anesthesia) avoid an incorrect intraoperative regulation of the cardiovascular system, leading to a reduced need for anesthesia drugs, particularly with regard to major surgeries [41], and therefore contribute to an active risk management. As a result, the anesthesia can be concluded more quickly and leads, due to continuous analgesia, to a stress shield and an earlier restoration of intestinal function. [41] The induction of such kind of anesthesia, however, requires additional measures and, just as the surgery itself, takes time, particularly when high quality standards are to be adhered to. In 2005, this wait time (anesthesia time alone (physician and supportive staff)) cost on average was EUR 2.50-3.00/min in Germany (depending on hospital size) [42]. For the surgical side (wait times of the surgical team), our calculations show [29] that the costs are similar. If these additional regional anesthesia methods, that are CTQ, are used in a more consistent manner, the overall time spent on the intensive care unit and in the hospital can be reduced significantly, leading to an increase in patient satisfaction [43] and profits [29].

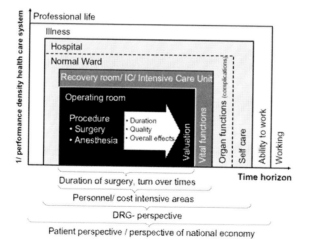

Figure 11. Treatment phases, locations, objectives, key figures and perspectives for performance in surgical medicine. Measures negatively impacting a core key figure (regional anesthesia → time between surgeries ↑) can favorable influence the next levels of treatment due to their overall effect (times for recovery room↓, intensive care unit↓, improved intestinal function, duration of hospitalization↓, illness↓, patient satisfaction↑) [4]

In this manner, the anesthesiologist can generate a benefit across treatment phases (Figure 11) that more than makes up for the surgeon's wait time [29]. Subsequently, a supportive process such as anesthesia can become a direct value driver, even if the time between surgeries (non-realized potential) becomes longer.

Therefore, we must ask if easy to obtain key figures such as (shorter) times between surgeries in the OR area are appropriate to adequately reflect the anesthesiologist's contribution to the overall process. Bender, the managing director of the first budget-responsible OR center in Germany, which is run as a service center, calculated that an 8-hour work day allows for no more than three surgical procedures >120 minutes, regardless of whether the time between patients is 20, 30 or 40 minutes [44]. Therefore, prolonging the anesthesia time by 5 minutes due to the use of regional anesthesia methods does not influence the process flow [29], since during 3 x 5 minute per day, it is not possible to do another surgery. Surgeries taking approx. 60 minutes are something else. Here, the difference between 30 or 40 minutes of time between surgeries may decide if 5 or 6 surgeries can be completed that day [44]. Therefore, the initially posed question as to whether the anesthesia induction takes too long, must always be considered in relation to the working methods of the surgical team.

It is undisputed that the supporting anesthesia process must strive for a more efficient workflow. Various key figures are also impacted by the severity of a case, so that this factor must be included in the evaluation in a separate manner. Since the time and effort spent increases exponentially in relationship to the severity of the case, the evaluation of the severity in accordance with the American Society of Anesthesiologists is squared in the evaluation (section 4).

One of the main goals in anesthesia is to minimize risk. Therefore, automated monitoring of unforeseen occurrences and undesired side effects, e.g., shivering, nausea, and vomiting, with the help of the routine database would be desirable. The so-called anesthesia observations are part of the scanner-readable anesthesia documentation used by the UHD. [36] The degree of discipline and honesty with which this documentation is provided varies significantly, so that the non-existence of documentation does not necessary mean that the anesthesiological care was top notch.

Conversely, a higher number of anesthesia observation documentations does not necessarily prove that the quality of the anesthesiologist's work is poor, merely because he documents more than the average anesthesiologist or actually does cause many unforeseen occurrences. Figure 12 shows how individual employees can influence the employer's observation window (key figure system) with regard to how the documents are affected in terms of a reporting bias [45]. On the opposite anesthesia observations such as existing fluid deficit and consequent hypotension followed by use of vasopressors or fluid infusion may vary seasonally or may be related to uncontrollable external factors such as weather.

Even though it is possible to gain information about the process by evaluating the anesthesia observations of *all* employees [46], a department-specific or individual-related evaluation is not valid because the reporting bias or external factors are not controllable (Figure 12) and therefore cannot be used directly to measure the performance of a senior staff member.

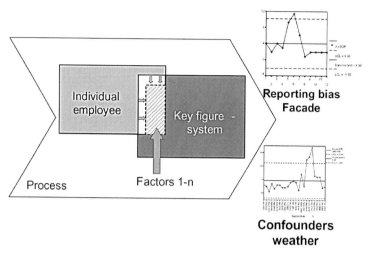

Figure 12. Employee involvement in the process and observer window into the process through the key figure system. Employee influence on the Johari arena [34] (arrows) due to reporting bias [45]. Employee controlled facade area striped.

BEHAVIOR THAT CANNOT BE PORTRAYED WITH A JUSTIFIABLE AMOUNT OF TIME AND EFFORT SPENT - SOFT KEY FIGURES

It is easy to evaluate performance in areas where it is quantifiable. The process from the performance to be evaluated to the key figure may be demanding and requires a considerable amount of scientific and technical work. The monitoring becomes especially difficult however, if it cannot be measured in the usual manner. Some examples of such characteristics are honesty, integrity, fairness, endurance, flexibility, creativity, the ability to communicate, selflessness, helpfulness, loyalty, ethical standards, exemplary leadership, obsession with power, effectiveness, strength of purpose, motivation, the ability to solve problems, the ability to work under pressure, behavior under pressure, and patient care.

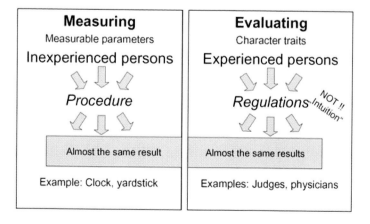

Figure 13. Measurement and evaluation as performance evaluation tools (own presentation as per [1]).

When evaluating these kinds of personality traits, the persons involved must be *evaluated* in addition to the computer-based key figure measurements. This evaluation is then ultimately incorporated into a usable evaluation. This inevitably leads to a discussion on objectivity, reliability, reproducibility, etc. According to Malik, measuring and evaluating do not necessarily oppose each other, but when used in accordance with correct procedures or regulations, lead to almost the same results, even when applied by several different users [1] (Figure 13).

Since the evaluations of the senior staff members by the employees over time are done by different employees, the subjectivity of the evaluation balances out in the long run, so that it can be assumed that the evaluation is objective after 3-4 evaluation rounds with 2-4 evaluators each.

To complete the character-related image of a senior staff member, Hilb suggests an overall evaluation by all stakeholders [18], e.g., the evaluation of the unit supervisor by employees, colleagues, superiors, customers and themselves, etc. But it is important to ask whether the benefit of a complete overview can justify the effort spent. If anything, such an overview evaluation should only relate to the CTQs of the senior staff member. [35] A complete evaluation by all stakeholders is an inappropriate control expenditure and does not fulfill the requirements. *"What do we have to control to be sufficiently confident that nothing goes seriously wrong?"* [1] Subsequently, this kind of evaluation is not appropriate for the task at hand. Additionally, it does not correspond to the meaningful control scope of 7±2 parameters. [30]

AGREEMENTS ON OBJECTIVES – EVALUATION MATRIX FOR THE CLINIC FOR ANESTHESIA/ UHD

Seventh question to predict victory or defeat:
The members of which army are more certain that their service will be
adequately rewarded and wrongdoing punished immediately?
Sunzi 500 A.D. [11]

The strategy, process, and organizational conditions outlined are summarized in a matrix that also takes the triangular relationship presented by Hilb (Figure 3) into consideration. The acceptance of a performance measurement system directly depends on the extent to which the employees feel that self-evaluation and the evaluation by the system are congruent. [13;18;21] Therefore, the evaluation matrix must be discussed with the employees and, depending on whether the performance is to be implemented within existing compensation systems or additional to it, has to be coordinated with the personnel department. At the same time, the simultaneous self-evaluation and evaluations by others can help uncover a future development potential of the senior staff member.

INTERNAL CLINIC CONCEPTS TO BE IMPLEMENTED

The matrix presented in Table 2 includes a 360 degree evaluation of the senior staff members doing clinical, research, or teaching work. It includes only a few CTQ key figures per area within the control scope [30]. The weightings of the individual fields of responsibility were taken from 2006 data used for the model calculations for senior staff members. This is how the case severity adjustment for pediatric anesthesia and the times for process time incentivization and the caps were established. The department-specific evaluation of the severity of a case (ASA^2) for 2006 was for example between 4.45 (trauma & orthopedics) and 7.58 (neurosurgery) points.

Table 2: Strategy supported 360 degree evaluation matrix for senior staff members of the anesthesia department of the UHD

Area	Function	Points	Evaluation
Patient care	Management task	2	Unit supervisor
		4	Senior physician
		6	Function of a leading physician
	Indiv. anesth. min.	0-9	1 for every started 10,000 min
	Ready for first surgery	3	Median ≤ 8:05 a.m.
		2	Median ≤ 8:10 a.m.
	Process sequence	3	ANT/IST < 1.4
		1	ANT/IST < 1.5
	Case severity	ASA^2	ø ASA-class^2 (+1 for pediatric surgery)
Scientific work	Publications	sum IF	cumul. impact factor (max. 10)
	Patents	3	
	Presentations*	0,25	per presentation (max. 3)
	Third party funds	0,1	procurement 1,000 € (max. 4)
Education, advanced training and continuing education	Student teaching	1	POL-Tutorshpi/CD/CC/Practicum
	internal continuing education	1-3	active internal continuing education involvement
	Clinic symposia	1-2	Organization/cooperation
Work method	Employee satisfaction	1-3	depending on survey results
	Reach objectives	1-3	Project completion
Miscellaneous**	Committees, admin.	1-2	

Senior physician (SP), Anesthesia time (ANT), Incision-Suture-time (IST), impact factor (IF), American Society of Anesthesiologists (ASA), Pediatric Surgery (PS), Problem oriented learning (POL), Course Director (CD), Course Coordinator (CC), Continuing Education (CE), * no poster, ** director's discretion

An internal, retraceable and equitable distribution can only be achieved, if different tasks are weighted in a balanced manner [18] that also encourage the willingness to rotate the unit supervisory responsibilities after an appropriate time period. [18] The corporate success equity of the matrix results from alignment to vision, mission, process, and structure. [10]

While the job market situation of the evaluation system for universities are a given, the effective amount to be paid out to the unit supervisor and thus the satisfaction of his individual needs depends on the available private liquidation pool. This pool may be comparable to those in the new German states, but is, aside from the already disadvantageous pay schedule for the Eastern states, a disadvantage in the competition for top performers. Accordingly, additional immaterial performance incentives must be offered. Employees will be given the opportunity to travel to symposia at the expense of the hospital if they are making a scientific contribution there. As an incentive to publish the data as an original paper (which benefits the clinic and the employees), the contribution presented at the symposium must, that same year, be developed into a manuscript ready for publication in order to justify approval for another trip to a symposium the following year, to be paid for by the hospital.

This version does not include individual caps and floors of the annual performance-related overall amount. [27] Explicit floors always make sense, if the performance related compensation constitutes a significant portion of the senior staff member's annual income to guarantee that staff member certain personal planning reliability. With regard to the case at hand, due to the pay scale-related basic financial security, this does generally not apply to most of the physicians paid in accordance with the TVÖD. In addition, a minimum amount of points is guaranteed by the consideration of the function in the matrix and the 360 degree perspective alone.

REPORTING/BENCHMARKING

Employees are provided information about the key data from the routine database [36] that was used to calculate the performance at the end of the year. I have developed an interim reporting system that primarily focuses on the strategy and incentivization-relevant key numbers, but it still needs to be automated. Only in this way can employees manage their objectives and the achievement of these objectives. We are striving for a monthly reporting system tied to the budget-relevant, department-specific figures (anesthesia minutes).

To be in a better position to estimate one's own performance, the departmental performance figures as benchmark are horizontally aligned in the form of an anonymous ranking of the senior staff members. In addition, since 2000 we participate in a benchmarking project among anesthesia departments in German university hospitals. To utilize the team approach within the operational units and to increase performance in a competitive manner, a quarterly report published clinic-wide about the departmental results, e.g., in the in-house magazine or the intranet, might also be of interest. When implementing a seamless IT structure, even a daily updated reporting system might be feasible.

CONCLUSION

Alignment of the employees´ workforce with the hospitals strategy, is a key issue for long term development and success. The level of hierarchy which in particular must be addressed is the middle management. This party decides over success or failure of any strategy driven activity of the top management by their degree of commitment and involvement. It is therefore indebatable, that hospitals to the same extent as successful companies, have to generate a WIN-WIN constellation upon success with their middle management, namely the Heads of Departments and the level of consultants.

Standard pay schedules within public healthcare systems are a major obstacle for introducing Management by objectives (MbO) tied to variable salary. If one hospital has managed this first step to pay on its own preference when having changed its legal form, a culture of professional MbO has to be implemented because it is the key link between company strategy and individual assignments and performance. The corporate objectives are, hence, expressed by the sum of the individual objectives of all employees which have to be defined *S.M.A.R.T.* and equitable in terms of internal distribution, corporate success, labor marked, and horizontal adjustment.

Time and money spent for performance measurement systems must clearly be weighed against improvement of corporate performance by MbO and key figures used must undoubtedly indicate what is intended to measure.

Overall, MbO bear the chance to improve the companies´ success to the degree individual salary is tied to the individual's contribution, lastly implementing entrepreneur way of thinking within each individual employee in the whole organization with the focus on critical to quality characteristics of the service.

REFERENCES

[1] Malik F. Führen Leisten Leben. 4 ed. Stuttgart: Deutsche Verlagsanstalt; 2000.

[2] Albrecht DM, Töpfer A. Erfolgreiches Changemanagement im Krankenhaus. 1 ed. Heidelberg: Springer; 2006.

[3] Böhlke R, Söhnle N, Viering S. Gesundheitsversorgung 2020. Frankfurt: Ernst & Young; 2005.

[4] Heller AR, Litz RJ, Koch T. Optimierung klinischer Behandlungspfade durch Regionalanästhesieverfahren. Anästh Intensivmed 2007;48:306-20.

[5] Michel S, Günther K-P, Joraschky P, Reichmann H, Koch T, Eberlein-Gonska M. Interdisziplinarität in der chronischen Schmerztherapie - Etablierung eines neuen fachübergreifenden Zentrums am Universitätsklinikum Dresden auf der Grundlage eines Vertrages zur integrierten Versorgung. Z Arztl Fortbild Qualitatssich 2007;101(3):165-71.

[6] Heller AR, Rössler S, Litz RJ, Stehr SN, Heller SC, Koch R, et al. Omega-3 fatty acids improve the diagnosis-related clinical outcome. Crit Care Med 2006 Apr;34(4):972-9.

[7] Hobbes T. Leviathan. London: 1651.

[8] Heller AR. Die Rechtsform eines Universitätsklinikums in der gegenwärtigen Haushaltslandschaft
- Erfahrungen aus 3 Jahren AöR am UKD, Chancen und Perspektiven. Vortrag: Workshop Prozesskontrolle und -Abbildung, Uniklinikum Halle 2005 Oct 13.

[9] Drucker PF. The Practice of Management. New York: Harper & Row; 1954.

[10] Chandler A. Strategy and Structure: Chapters in the history of industrial enterprise. New York: Doubleday; 1962.

[11] Sunzi W. Die Kunst des Krieges. München: Droemer Knaur; 2001.

[12] Drucker PF. Das Geheimnis effizienter Führung. Harvard Businesss Manager 2005;(3):7-14.

[13] Kaplan R, Norton D. The Balanced Scorecard. Translating Strategy Into Action. 1 ed. Boston: Harvard Business School Press; 1996.

[14] European Foundation for Quality Management. Excellence einführen. Brüssel: EFQM; 2003.

[15] Eberlein-Gonska M. Zielvereinbarungsgespräche. Dresden: Universitätsklinikum, internes Verfahren; 2002.

[16] Beitz H. Zielvereinbarungen. Das Handbuch für den Vorgesetzten, Loseblattsammlung.Bonn: Fachverlag für Recht und Führung; 2001.

[17] Ackermann M. Zielvereinbarung mit Erfolgshonorierung. Das Handbuch für den Vorgesetzten, Loseblattsammlung.Bonn: Fachverlag für Recht und Führung; 2001.

[18] Hilb M. Integriertes Personalmanagement. 14 ed. München: Luchterhand; 2005.

[19] Gauss CF. Werke. Göttingen: Dieterich; 1863.

[20] Svoboda V. Zielsicher zum Erfolg - Leistungs- und erfolgsabhängige Vergütung auf der Basis von Zielvereinbarungen in der Deutschen Bank. In: Bundgard W, Kohnke O, editors. Zielvereinbarungen erfolgreich umsetzen.Wiesbaden: Gabler Verlag; 2000.

[21] Baum HG, Coenenberg AG, Günther T. Strategisches Controlling. 4 ed. Stuttgart: Schäffer-Poerschel; 2007.

[22] Heller AR. Kosten- Nutzen- Relation von Fast Track Chirurgie. Vortrag: 123 Deutscher Chirurgenkongress, Berlin 2006 May 5.

[23] Braun JP, Walter M, Kuhly R, Lein M, Everslage K, Hansen D, et al. Clinical Pathways und Diagnosis-Related Groups: Die Anästhesiologie als Schnittstellenfach . Anaesthesiologie & Intensivmedizin 2003;44:637-46.

[24] Siegmund F, Berry M, Martin J, Geldner G, Bauer M, Bender HJ, et al. Entwicklungsstand im OP-Management - Eine Analyse in deutschen Krankenhäusern im Jahr 2005. Anaesthesiologie & Intensivmedizin 2006;47(12):743-50.

[25] Bauer M, Forum Ökonomie und QM. MultiCenterStudie: Benchmark Prozesszeiten. Ergebnispräsentation Deutsche Anästhesiekongress Leipzig 2006.

[26] Heller AR, Koch T, Töpfer A. Phoenix - Führungs- und Personalentwicklungsworkshop an der Klinik für Anästhesie und Intensivtherapie am Uniklinikum Dresden. laufende Projektarbeit 2007 Mar 12.

[27] Hofbauer H, Winkler B. Das Mitarbeitergespräch als Führungsinstrument. 3 ed. München: Hanser; 2004.

[28] Koch T, Heller AR, Rasche S. Jahresbericht der Klinik für Anästhesiologie und Intensivtherapie am Uniklinikum Dresden 2005/ 2006. Aachen: Shaker Verlag; 2007.

[29] Heller AR, Litz RJ, Wiessner D, Dammann C, Weissgerber R, Hakenberg OW, et al. Betriebswirtschaftliche Auswirkungen der thorakalen Epiduralanästhesie am Beispiel der G-DRG M01B, OPS-301 5-604.0. Anaesthesist 2005 Dec;54(12):1176-85.

[30] Miller GA. The magic number seven plus / minus two. Psychol Rev 1956;63:81-2.

[31] Ansorg J, Diemer M, Schleppers A, Heberer J, von Eiff W. OP- Management. Berlin: Medizinisch Wissenschaftliche Verlagsgesellschaft; 2006.

[32] Lay R. Führen durch das Wort. 5 ed. München: 2002.

[33] Köllner V. Gibt es ein Selbst in der Verhaltenstherapie? Psychotherapie im Dialog 2004;(3):231-5.

[34] Luft J, Ingham H. The Johari Window, a graphic model for interpersonal relations. Los Angeles: University of California; 1955.

[35] Töpfer A. Six Sigma. 3 ed. Berlin: Springer; 2004.

[36] Heller AR, Böhme G. Routinedatenbank für Anästhesieleistungen/ UKD. AnDok-Anästhesiedatenbank, DataPec Pliezhausen 2005.

[37] Heller AR. Möglichkeiten und Grenzen eines Prozesscontrollings im Krankenhaus. Dresden: Dresden International University; 2007.

[38] Klöss T. Kennzahlen im OP-Management. Vortrag: Fortbildungsreihe OP-ManagerBDA/ BDC/ Malik Management Zentrum St Gallen 2005.

[39] Schönherr R. Prozesscontrolling im Krankenhaus. 1 ed. Dresden: TUDpress; 2006.

[40] Heller AR, Koch T. Weiterbildung Anästhesie. Stuttgart: Thieme; 2006.

[41] Heller AR, Litz RJ, Djonlagic I, Manseck A, Koch T, Wirth MP, et al. Kombinierte Anasthesie mit Epiduralkatheter. Eine retrospektive Analyse des perioperativen Verlaufs bei Patienten mit radikalen Prostatektomien. Anaesthesist 2000 Nov;49(11):949-59.

[42] Berry M, Martin J, Geldner G, Iber T, Bauer M, Bender HJ, et al. Analyse der IST-Kosten Anästhesie in deutschen Krankenhäusern - Bezugsjahr 2005. Anaesthesiologie & Intensivmedizin 2007;48(3):140-6.

[43] Heller AR, Horter M, Horter S, Koch T. Quality of anaesthesia - a patient´s view. Eur J Anaesthesiology 2003;20(Supplement 30):-4.

[44] Bender HJ, Waschke K, Schleppers A. Are turnover times a measure of effective operating room management. Anästh Intensivmed 2004;9:529-35.

[45] Greenhalgh T. How to Read a Paper: The Basics of Evidence-Based Medicine. 3 ed. Oxford: Blackwell Publishing; 2006.

[46] Heller AR, Katzer M, Knoth H, Koch T. Nutzen und Risiken der richtliniengetreuen Verwendung von Succinylcholin - Eine Kohortenstudie. Abstractband Deutscher Anästhesiekongress (DAC) 2006. Ref Type: Abstract

ISBN 978-1-60692-307-8

Chapter 4

SHARED MENTAL MODELS AND TEAM LEARNING: CONSEQUENCES FOR IMPROVING PATIENT SAFETY

Piet van den Bossche[1], Myrthe Akkermans[2],Wim Gijselaers[3] and Mien Segers[4]

[1]Department of Educational Development and Educational Research, Faculty of Economics and Business Administration, Maastricht University
[2]Novius Consultancy, Amersfoort, the Netherlands
[3]Department of Educational Development and Educational Research, Faculty of Economics and Business Administration, Maastricht University
[4]Department of Educational Development and Educational Research, Faculty of Economics and Business Administration, Maastricht University

ABSTRACT

Research on minimizing error in medicine so far focused largely on individual's expertise in terms of the organization of knowledge, diagnostic ability, and technical skills, as significant components of medical practice. However, as medicine became a complex profession functioning in multi-disciplinary teams became part of the daily job of health professionals. Unfortunately, we have limited understanding about the consequences of team-work for team performance and patient safety. The present chapter describes how research insights from business on team work can provide enhanced understanding of team work in medicine and its consequences for patient safety. It places analysis of development of shared mental models at the core to understand how multi-professional teams function. Based on a series of empirical studies we demonstrate how understanding team behavior can improve patient safety.

INTRODUCTION

Medicine has undergone an unparalleled change over the past century with respect to the development of knowledge bases, introduction of sophisticated technologies and control systems, and its positive contributions to societal health and welfare. This has had tremendous consequences for the schooling of medical students, the continuous training of health professionals, the organization and finance of health care, and the design of complex medical hospitals delivering top-class care. It goes beyond saying that next to its huge success in improving health, legal claims against individual doctors and hospitals have increased as well. This underlines the need for research on minimizing human error in medicine. Most of the research so far focused largely on individual's expertise in terms of the organization of knowledge, diagnostic ability, and technical skills, as significant components of medical practice. However, as medicine became a complex profession, incorporating the input and collaboration of a wide range of disciplines, functioning in multi-disciplinary teams became part of the daily job of health professionals. Unfortunately, while medicine went through an exponential increase of its knowledge base contributing to improved understanding diagnosis, treatment and prevention of human disease, these increases have not equaled our understanding about the limitations of this team-work and its consequences for team performance and patient safety. The present chapter describes research on team work that is quite different from medicine – business – yet it can provide enhanced understanding of team work in medicine and its consequences for patient safety. We will examine the nature of team-learning processes and its effects on team performance. Next we will address the question how our insights can be applied to medicine.

TEAMWORK

Organizations increasingly turn to team-based working to contend with the growing complexity of the environment in which they operate [1,2]. It is argued that teams have the potential to offer greater adaptability, productivity and creativity than any one individual can offer and provide more complex, innovative and comprehensive solutions to organizational problems [2,3]. Teams can bring together people who have a variety of backgrounds, points of view, education, and/or expertise. Therefore, it is assumed that such teams can bring multiple perspectives to bear on a problem, which allows for the rich problem conceptualization required to solve complex problems [3,4]. However, both experiences and empirical research demonstrate that teams are not easily implemented and that the creation of a team of skilled members does not ensure success; teamwork does not just happen [2,5].

Recent research by Amy Edmondson and her co-workers [6,7,8] provides a case in point. They analyzed in a series of studies why hospitals make mistakes, how the introduction of new technologies in cardiac surgery-teams can provide a hazard to patients, and how different leadership styles affect the performance of nursing teams. These studies share in common that they examined how various kinds of hospital teams (nursing, top-tier cardiac surgery teams) are prone for making medical mistakes. Her field study in 16 hospitals with Bohmer and Pisano [7] provides an interesting example of how patient safety is affected by the introduction of new technologies for cardiac surgery: Minimally Invasive Cardiac Surgery (MICS). In her view organizations develop routines around the use of existing technologies that allow teams to perform in a stable way. However, adaptation of new technologies requires that teams have to learn about new procedures, are required to unlearn routines, and have to acquire new understanding and technical knowledge. Next, teams may have to change their communication and social behavior when using new technology. Her study demonstrated that successful teams – with respect to implementing new technologies for cardiac surgery – were teams capable to develop learning practices. The nature of social processes within the surgery teams determined whether these teams could adapt the new technology. Leadership was essential to establish a climate of trust and psychological safety necessary for learning MICS [7]: "Existing routines and status relationships in the context of cardiac surgery presented powerful barriers to implementing MICS [p. 707]." They also found that changing communication patterns within surgery teams was crucial to work with this new technology: "The kind of top-down, one-way communication that was problematic in learning MICS can be essential to saving lives in critical moments during conventional cardiac surgery. [p. 710]".

Edmondson's work was focused on identifying characteristics of the work context – e.g., team characteristics and team learning processes – and its effects on performance of medical teams. Lingard and her colleagues [9] researched the nature of communication taking place within surgery teams and its effects on medical error. They found that ineffective team communication can be at the root of medical error [9]. Teams that demonstrated poor communication were characterized by a lack of standardization and team integration. Typically, poor teams failed to analyze a case in-depth before surgery took place. Another typical behavior of poor teams was that decision-making took place without all relevant team members being present. She concluded that "we have found that these failures are based in strikingly simple factors: communication is too late to be effective, content is not consistently complete and accurate, key individuals are excluded, and issues are left unresolved until the point of urgency [p. 332]." One of her recommendations was that OR-teams should try to work with checklists, following the examples from aviation.

Aviation has developed substantial knowledge and management practices for dealing with safety issues. It provides many insights on how to improve flight safety by improved training of pilots, development of clear procedures for air traffic control, management of aircraft maintenance, communication within cockpits, and certification of people and equipment. The question may be raised whether insights from aviation can be transferred to medicine. Davies [10] points out that in aviation many accidents can be explained by causes of human error and not by malfunctioning equipment or poor maintenance. In more than two thirds of all aviation accidents problems in communication, teamwork, leadership, and decision making played a decisive role. In those cases the main cause of error lied in human error and not in failures with equipment or lack of technical competence. This finding resulted in a substantial body of research addressing the problem of how flight crews allocate resources in times of stress [11]. Nowadays, training pilots includes – next to technical, navigation and aviation competencies – competencies that acknowledge the importance of interpersonal behavior. In aviation this is generally known as crew resource management (CRM). Nowadays, airlines have invested in CRM to promote teamwork in the cockpit and to reduce errors. CRM has been accepted by aviation industry as a standard practice for training cockpit crews. It puts its emphasizes on training team work processes, and adds on the traditional focus of training individuals in developing individual skills and knowledge. At the core of CRM lies the idea that teams should develop complementary skills and knowledge resulting in a common set of performance goals and standards. Furthermore CRM underscore the need to embed CRM practices at the core of organizational activities [11]. As a consequence, pilot work is considered to be a team-work activity requiring particular attention for training team skills and team understanding.

Despite the evident success of CRM in aviation, it has been difficult to transfer the lessons learned from aviation to non-aviation domains. Until the beginning of 2000 only few practices were identified using insights from CRM. Davies [10] is one of the few who attempted to apply CRM to anesthesiology. Despite the availability of few CRM practices outside aviation, an increasing amount of research has become available that applies lessons learned from CRM in other areas. Next, we have witnessed an increasing amount of research on team-learning processes and its applications in many areas that require team work [e.g., industrial design, engineering, management, and nursing). Finally, in our consultancy and practice the authors have observed increasing attention for the outcomes of team-learning research and its applications in business and medicine. For example, the medical schools of the University of Dresden (Germany), and Maxima Hospital Veldhoven (the Netherlands), apply various insights from team-learning research – which lie at the heart of CRM – on team-work setting in training of anesthetics and gynecology. In both organizations they try to reduce error by incorporating insights from CRM and team-learning research in the training of medical professionals.

The present chapter presents results from team-learning research in business that are also of great value to gain insight in critical success-factors for team-work in medicine. We will focus on the notion of team-learning processes as the key for understanding and improving team processes. In particular, attention will be paid to the idea of shared mental models as an instrument to understand and assess the development of team cognition and team performance. In our view understanding how shared mental models are developed is at the core of understanding team-learning processes and its consequences for team performance. Whether team performance is understood as avoidance of (medical) error, or in the creation of new products, or in making decisions about new business strategies, doesn't matter. In our view understanding how professionals make decisions requires understanding of communication between professionals and how professionals share their thoughts and insights about the problems at hand.

TEAM LEARNING PROCESSES: A ROAD TO SHARED MENTAL MODELS

A team is more than a group of people in the same space; physical or virtual. In recent years, increasing attention has been devoted to the social bases of cognition whereby research on information processing and its consequences for professional decision-making has taken into consideration how social processes in groups and teams affect performance.

Teams are increasingly being employed to discuss and manage complex problems. Organizations rely on these teams to deal with a fast-changing and highly competitive environment. Teams are ascribed high potential since they can bring together people with different experience and expertise. It is generally assumed that making decisions in such teams enhances the likelihood that the decisions will not only incorporate multiple perspectives but that new levels of understandings will develop [12]. However, research and practice shows that this potential effectiveness is not always reached. Research has revealed cases in which large variation in group-work interaction and performance is encountered between teams that seem not to differ in composition and assigned task [13]. This research indicates that fruitful collaboration is not merely a case of putting people with relevant knowledge together. This outcome has been found in many domains ranging from kids working in groups at schools [14], business professionals working in product-development teams [15], or medical professionals working in operating rooms [7,9]. So the question can be raised why good team work is so difficult to accomplish.

Understanding how individuals make decisions lies at the heart of cognitive research. It has established that knowledge structures affect information processing in predictable ways. The importance of domain-specific knowledge has especially been identified as the prime determinant of excellent performance across many different expertise domains such as medicine, engineering, or management [16,17,18,19]. This area of research concentrates on how individuals process information, how they assess and interpret situations, and how they solve problems. With the increasing interest in teamwork, the question of how these individual cognitions become integrated and coordinated at the inter-individual level becomes of central interest [20]. In this perspective, the construction of shared mental model (i.e., shared conception of the problem) lies at the heart of collaboration [14,21]. This implies that studying group performance requires an analysis of the socio-cognitive processes within the group. As Langfield-Smith [22] has argued, to understand how collective knowledge structures are formed, it is a basic requirement that one must understand the interaction between cognition and social processes.

Our Department of Educational Development and Educational Research at Maastricht University conducted a series of studies to analyze how people from different backgrounds work together on a series of tasks, and how collaboration and learning behavior in teams are related to team performance. The foundational conceptual framework of our studies was shaped by an input-mediator-process-output framework [23]. This framework is depicted in Figure 1. It proposes that crucial mediators for effective teamwork can be found in the development of shared mental models, achievement of a beneficial interpersonal context, and engagement in learning behavior. The latter, learning behavior, grasps essential socio-cognitive processes, the former two, shared mental models and interpersonal context are emergent states, respectively cognitive and social by nature. Concerning the input variables, we focused on diversity in composition of the team. For measuring the team output, we took a broad approach regarding team effectiveness including performance, viability and learning.

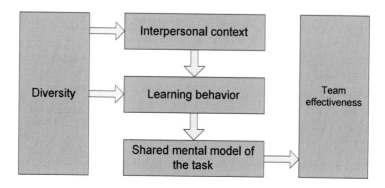

Figure 1. Team effectiveness framework.

Shared Mental Model of the Task

Several researchers describe team behavior and explain team performance from the cognitive standpoint of shared mental models [24] (see Figure 1). It has been argued that the shared mental model of the task integrates and coordinates the perspectives available in the team and enables the team to have a complex and rich understanding of the task environment [25], resulting in better problem-solving performance.

Shared mental models assure that all team members are solving the same problem and help exploit the cognitive capabilities of the entire team. This enables the team to have a complex and rich understanding of the task environment [26,27].

Team Learning Behaviors

In our view the development of shared mental models is more than a cognitive process of integrating and coordinating perspectives. We stress the relevance of socio-cognitive processes that serve as mediators promoting the development of shared mental models. We define these socio-cognitive processes as 'learning behaviors' (see Figure 1), stressing how characteristics of the behaviors interact with knowledge building processes that lead to shared mental models [14]. Achieving a shared mental model is not only a matter of understanding each other's representation (mutual understanding), but also of accepting and incorporating each other's ways of seeing (mutual agreement) [28,29]. To determine the team interactions that can be considered as team learning behavior we refer to the processes of construction, co-construction and constructive conflict to reach the necessary mutual understanding and agreement.

First, meaning or understanding needs to be *(co-)constructed*. This process starts when one of the team members inserts meaning by describing the problem situation and how to deal with it, hereby tuning in to fellow team-members. These processes of construction of meaning can evolve into collaborative construction (co-construction), which is a mutual process of building meaning by refining, building on, or modifying the original offer in some way [30]. This can lead to 'new' meanings that were not previously available to the group.

Second, agreement needs to be established about the (co-)constructed understandings.

It is not sufficient that the inserted meanings are clarified and that there is mutual understanding. They must also be accepted before they form the basis for action [29]. However, team members may diverge in their interpretation and tackle the situation from another point of view or perspective. This can lead to a further elaboration through the negotiation of the different meanings. The team will only benefit if divergence in meaning leads to deep-level processing of the diverse information and viewpoints in the team. Through this negotiation by argument and clarification, this is constructive conflict, the team works towards a convergence of meaning in order to reach shared mental models.

Interpersonal Context

In our view it is essential to identify social conditions under which teams make the effort to reach shared mental models. Viewing teamwork as reaching shared mental models, and thus as social, stresses the need to take into account the social context in which these processes take place. Therefore, it is crucial to focus on emerging team-level beliefs about the relations between the team members; in other words beliefs about the interpersonal context (see Figure 1). Shared beliefs of the team-characteristics emerge in groups from the interaction between the team members [31]. It is supposed that these interpersonal beliefs form a context that influences team learning behaviors. We identified a number of powerful group-level beliefs which potentially affect the learning behavior in teams: psychological safety, task cohesion, potency and interdependence. It was hypothesized that teams will engage in learning behavior when specific social conditions are realized.

First, there has to be shared task cohesion. This task cohesion refers to the shared commitment among members to achieve a goal that requires the collective efforts of the team [32]. Task cohesion will be positively associated with learning behavior, because high task motivation shows the existence of shared goals and the motivation to strive for it.

Further they have to believe that they need each other for dealing with this task: there needs to be perceived interdependence. Interdependence refers on the one hand to the interconnections between tasks such that the performance of one piece of work depends on the completion of other pieces of work and on the other hand to the extent to which personal benefits depend on successful goal attainment by other team members [33] It has been shown that this leads to a shared responsibility and influences the level of cooperative social interaction in teams [34].

Third, the team believes they will not be rejected for proposing ideas (team psychological safety). Psychological safety facilitates learning behavior because it alleviates excessive concern about others' reactions to actions that have the potential for embarrassment, which learning behaviors often have [6].

Finally, they believe that the team is capable of using this new information to generate useful results (team potency). This is the belief of the team members that the group can be effective [35]. Potency fosters a team's confidence.

Diversity

The potential of teams is for a large part due to teams bringing together people who have a variety of backgrounds, points of view, education, and/or expertise. These resources make it possible that teams can bring multiple perspectives to bear on a problem, which can allow a rich problem conceptualization required to solve complex problems [3,4,36]. For that reason, it is necessary to consider the ways in which diversity (see Figure 1) influences the mediators. As a consequence one has to deal explicitly with the issue of a diverse composition of the team by depicting the informational and social category diversity of the teams.

SOCIAL AND COGNITIVE FACTORS DRIVING TEAMWORK

Van den Bossche, Gijselaers, Segers and Kirschner [37] found evidence supporting their claim that both interpersonal and socio-cognitive processes have to be taken into account to understand the formation of shared mental models, resulting in higher perceived team performance. Interdependence, task cohesion, psychological safety, and group potency, as aspects of the interpersonal context, appeared to be crucial for the engagement in team learning behaviors. The identified team learning behaviors, in turn, give rise to shared mental models. Also it was found that shared mental models are an important factor to understand perceived team effectiveness. One of the most striking findings was that development of shared mental models was largely dependent on building a climate of group trust or psychological safety. This finding confirmed earlier findings of Edmondson [6] about her research in hospitals showing that team performance was strongly related to psychological safety.

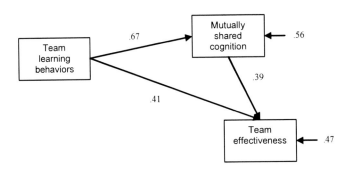

Figure 2. Path Analysis Cognition & Collaboration [adapted from 37].

Van den Bossche and co-workers [37] demonstrated in their study the importance of team learning behaviors and shared mental models (i.e., mutually shared cognition) for team effectiveness. Shared mental models can be seen as a primary and most profound learning outcome. In turn, this shared mental model is identified as a part of the basis on which team effectiveness is built: it plays an important role in the total effectiveness of the team. The relation between the team learning behaviors and team effectiveness is only partially mediated by shared mental models. Figure 2 present the paths between the variables as analyzed in our research. Coefficients represent Beta-weights which can be interpreted as standardized partial correlations. It makes clear that team learning behaviors have a relatively strong connection with shared mental models. Next, shared cognition serves as mediator between team learning and team effectiveness.

The final analysis in this study focused on integrating the identified input, process and output variables. The question was how team beliefs affected team-learning behaviors, which in turn determined shared mental models and team effectiveness.

Figure 3 shows how team effectiveness could be explained by the direct effect of shared mental models and the indirect effects of the input and process variables. We found strong evidence that team-learning behaviors do not take place just by putting people together. Interpersonal context needs to be taken into account to understand the engagement of team members to coordinate their understanding. The identified aspects such as interdependence, task cohesion, psychological safety and group potency turned out to be crucial for the engagement in team learning behavior in teams, which in turn give rise to shared mental models, in turn leading to higher perceived team effectiveness.

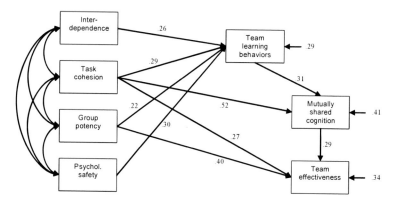

Figure 3. Integrative model (adapted from 37).

In an additional series of studies Van den Bossche [38] further elaborated on developing a detailed understanding of how social processes in teams interact with cognitive processes and team performance. He conducted these studies in a variety of contexts, ranging from student teams working in business simulators to established professional teams working in a company setting. The issue was whether the complex mechanisms between social aspects of teams on one hand could be understood to explain the cognitive processes underlying collaboration. This kind of research is relevant for many settings where people work together in teams. Understanding these processes may indeed help us to understand why some teams are better than others, but even more important, it may provide tools to understand why some teams are likely to run into more problems than others. As the work of Edmondson [6,7,8] and Lingard [9] has shown, understanding the social nature of team work in health care teams may indeed result in improved understanding why some OR-teams face difficulties in learning to work with new technologies and operating procedures, or why some nursing teams report more medical errors than others.

TEAM LEARNING AND CONFLICT

Van den Bossche's second empirical study questioned the role of team conflict and the development of shared mental models in teams [38]. This study shed light on a complex relation between team learning behaviors and the development of shared mental models in a team. We were especially interested in the impact of conflict on team-learning behavior. Conflict can be understood in its classical meaning of conflict between people (personal conflict), or conflict about the tasks required to be done (task conflict). However, conflict can also be defined in terms of differences in point of view inviting people to reexamine their points of view, to clarify meaning, or to bring in additional arguments in a discussion. This type of conflict is defined as constructive conflict. It has been found that constructive conflict is a critical determinant in the process of building shared mental models; only if there is a critical stance regarding each other contributions, if there is thorough consideration of each other ideas and comments, and if team members address differences in opinion and can speak freely, there will be construction of a shared mental model.

To investigate this in-depth, we used a business simulator which puts people under pressure to make decisions every 60 seconds [39,40]. Next, the task environment is highly complex. People work together in teams of 2 – 3 persons, requiring constant monitoring of data, coordination between members, and explicit analysis of the situation at hand. Failure to do so may result in a "business crash". The business simulator is run on a PC. Teams run the risk of information overload because the information about their business is complex and changes every 60 seconds. Teams have the availability about many distinctly different business functions. As a consequence constantly changing business intelligence data, and market data may cause stress and conflict between team members. Coordination of action, information sharing, and collaboration are necessary to avoid information overload, or losing the overview of market developments. Communication between team members is essential to develop shared understanding of the situation their business is facing. Stress may occur as soon as the manager of the simulator builds in a sudden crisis that may have disruptive effects on business routines and market behavior.

The use of this simulator allows us to study team behavior in a complex and constantly changing environment. It offers a challenging environment that shares basic characteristics with the situation management teams are confronted with, and at the same time it provides a controlled research setting for examining critical factors influencing team learning and effectiveness [39]. Additionally, the simulation game offers objective measures of team performance, presenting the effect of team decisions on the mean equity and goodwill of the company the team was managing.

Our research conducted in this setting [38] demonstrated that the development of a shared mental model results in substantially better team performance. In this particular case, the results of a company increase if the management team has developed a higher level of shared mental model of their environment. Moreover, the development of shared mental model mediates the relation between team learning behavior and (objective) business performance. Indicating that team learning has its effect on actual team performance through the development of a shared cognitive framework to comprehend the situation. Constructive conflict was found to be of major importance for developing shared mental models.

Now that we felt that we captured essential variables to explain team performance by measurement of social and cognitive processes, it was important to validate our model in settings characterized by diversity in team composition. Research on team diversity has become prominent because in professional practice people from various professional background work together in handling complex problems. In medicine this is the case for multi-professional OR-teams (junior surgeon, senior surgeon, nurse, anesthesiologist), in business for corporate boards of large companies (accounting, finance, marketing, management), and in engineering for the design of complex equipment. Diversity is not only represented by diversity in education and training, but also by gender, age, status, culture etc.

Despite the potential of multi-professional teams, people with different professional training, skills, experiences, and orientations are likely to have divergent perspectives and this can create conflict [41]. Conflict, as one of the most researched intermediate processes between diversity attributes of teams and the performance of the teams, signifies the experience of disagreements between team members [42,43]. This may hinder the development of a shared mental model. But if teams are able to harness this knowledge and are capable of constructively dealing with different points of view, they may have a greater wealth of knowledge to draw upon [44]. Constructive conflict refers to the learning behaviors of teams that enable them to integrate the available perspectives [45] and foster a shared mental model relevant to the task at hand. It is important to consider that processes as constructive conflict do not occur in a vacuum, but are influenced by the social context in which they take place [46]. In this light, researchers have pointed to the importance of a climate of trust in teams [47]. Alike, Edmondson's [6] research has established a relation between psychological safety in the team and productive team processes.

Again we examined the development of shared mental models as a crucial mechanism in explaining team effectiveness. Also we put forward psychological safety as important variable in the interpersonal context, grasping if the environment is characterized by trust and open for diverse viewpoints. The results of the analysis indicated that constructive conflict, contrary to task conflict, is positively related to performance. These results added to the evidence that the potential benefits of diversity are realized through the cross-fertilization of ideas that occurs through team learning behaviors and fail to support a role for task conflict in mediating the relationship between diversity and team performance [42]. Moreover, in the educational setting, the results indicate that constructive conflicts give rise to shared mental models. This underpins the idea that constructive conflicts bring to bear the potential of the diversity of knowledge available; it leads to the integration of perspectives in a shared mental model.

The studies by Van den Bossche [37,38] identified a number of powerful group-level beliefs which affect the learning behavior in teams: psychological safety, cohesion, potency and interdependence. It was found that interpersonal beliefs play an important role in fostering fruitful learning behavior. Moreover, it appears that psychological safety strongly promotes behaviors contributing significantly to team effectiveness. In general, our research demonstrated that interpersonal beliefs substantially add to the understanding of effective teamwork and particularly in understanding the emergence of productive team learning behavior. Team learning behaviors do not take place just by putting people together. The beliefs about the interpersonal context need to be taken into account to understand the engagement of team members to coordinate their understanding.

In our view this research demonstrates the importance of understanding how people belief they relate to each other. We feel that the 'cognitive side' of teamwork seems a reflection of the 'social picture' of the team. The way teams develop shared understanding of a problem at hand, and what needs to be done can not only be explained by understanding individual cognition. This makes it necessary to broaden the scope of research on error in medicine, and pay attention as well to the level of teams. It is crucial to understand the social process underlying cognitive performance of a team. Our studies demonstrated in a consistent fashion the importance of building a climate of psychological safety as a key requirement before any effective team learning behavior can take place. This finding is in line with Edmondson's [6,7,8] research about nursing teams and cardiac surgery teams demonstrating that the amount of medical errors reported or observed was associated with social processes in the team. She found as well that building a climate of psychological safety is essential for any team that wants to minimize error, or to improve performance. These findings concur with Davies' idea [10] that *"with the increased emphasis on care by teams has come a change in the nature of risks associated with medical practice. Although always a high-risk activity, the origin of the risk has shifted. Many of the problems now seen in medicine occur with difficulties in teamwork and communication. These interface issues have been shown to occur in the OR as well in aviation (p 269)."*

STRESS AND ITS IMPACT ON TEAM-DECISION MAKING

The studies described above provide a clear understanding of the importance of socio-cognitive processes in teams and its effects on team performance. They can also help us in the design of team training, and development of procedures to encourage improvement, and avoid poor team performance. But before paying attention to these issues, we want to take our analysis on team performance one step further. Now that we know about variables affecting team performance, we were interested in conditions that invoke stress within teams and its consequences for the shared cognition and team performance. This kind of research is especially relevant for teams that deal with complex work situations, cope with risk and uncertainty, and have to do their job under time pressure. Typically, this kind of situations may occur in medicine, aviation, air-traffic control, nuclear power plants, etc.

Davies [10] argues that in health care doctors, nurses, and paramedical personnel are taught they are to function without error. Flawless performance is considered to happen automatically when individual's knowledge and skills are up-to-date. However, Edmondson and co-workers [6], and Lingard and her colleagues [9] have shown that teams are more than a collection of individuals. A systems approach is necessary to understand why under certain conditions teams fail or realize success. Perceived time pressure and perceived task complexity are variables that may disrupt flawless decision-making in health-care teams. They may in particular affect development of shared cognition because high time pressure and high task complexity may cause a cognitive overload for a health care team, may increase social tension between members, and reduce the individual's capacity to understand the patient's problem. It is known from research that health care workers fail to recognize conditions that may limit their abilities due to fatigue, or other stress factors. For that reason, it is relevant to examine how stress factors such as time pressure and task complexity affect development of shared cognition and performance.

Empirical studies have shown that functionally diverse teams can be more innovative [48], can develop clearer strategies [49], can better respond to competitive threats and are quicker to implement types of organizational change than homogeneous teams. However, having access to resources in the group is not sufficient for successful performance if the group fails to use them effectively [50]. In order to adequately solve problems and make decisions, individual cognitions within a team need to be integrated and coordinated at the intra-individual level.

Akkermans' [51] research provides a case in point. She conducted a study- using the business simulator described above - hypothesizing that time pressure and task complexity is related to team performance through the team learning behaviors and the sharedness of the team mental model. In her view teams are challenged to integrate different knowledge, skills, information and perspectives in order to reach a shared interpretation of the environment/task with which the team is dealing [25]. Success is not only a function of the individual's talents and the available resources, but also the processes that team members use to in their interaction to accomplish a certain task. The processes that convert the inputs of individual team members to outcomes aimed at organizing work to reach collective (shared) goals are called team learning behaviors [23]. We examined the relation of perceived time pressure and task complexity with these team learning behaviors and the development of shared mental models. Figure 4 contains the conceptual model of our research on time pressure and task complexity. It builds further upon Van den Bossche's work [37, 38, 45]. Perceptions of task complexity and time pressure are considered as a condition that may invoke stress in teams, which in turn influences their capacity to learn and develop shared understanding.

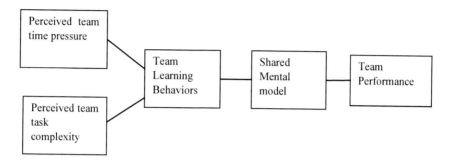

Figure 4. Perceptions of Time Pressure & Task Complexity and its Effects on Shared Mental Models and Team Performance.

Perceived Task Complexity

The team's ability to recognize the expertise of its members often can be vital to their effectiveness and performance. Research of Baumann, Bonner and Reeshad [52] has shown that some groups are very effective in the identification of team member expertise while other groups show to be very ineffective in this identification. This often appears to be a function of the complexity of the tasks that are performed by each group. It is important to note that task complexity is not the same as task difficulty. Task complexity is an objective characteristic of the task which affects perceived difficulty together with the individual characteristics (expertise level). While task complexity is an objective characteristic of the task, task difficulty is a subjective task characteristic. An example will be given to illustrate this difference. Imagine a certain task like doing a task in which one has to make decisions about certain variables. The task in which you are attending to one variable is easier than the task in which you have to attend to two variables, and this again is easier than the task in which you have to attend to three. Everyone would agree on this. When a task has the same complexity level for all people, for example five variables to make decisions about, there is no difference in task complexity. However, one person can find the task more difficult to perform than another. In this case we talk about perceived task complexity or task difficulty which is determined by the task complexity and the expertise level of the person involved.

Time Pressure

Time constraints have an important influence on team processes. Before we start explaining this influence, it needs to be mentioned that limited time or time pressure, like task complexity, can be objective or subjective. An example will be given to illustrate this difference: when a team has to perform a certain task in one minute, this time pressure is higher than the same task in which they have two minutes time to perform. Everyone would agree that the one minute task has a higher time pressure than the two minute task; this is the objective time pressure. Subjective time pressure is the time pressure that people perceive when doing a task of the same objective time pressure; when two persons perform the same task and they both have one minute, one person can perceive a really high time pressure while the other person has enough time to perform the task successfully. In our research we focused on subjective time pressure, because the students who participated in this study had to perform a complex task at the same objective time level, so they did not differ in objective time pressure but only in the subjective, perceived time pressure. Whether it is real or self-imposed, time pressure is one of the most important enemies of integrative negotiation because it increases cognitive closure. With cognitive closure people stop considering multiple alternatives, engage in shallow rather than thorough systematic information processing and rely more on cognitive heuristics when making decisions and solving problems [53], which means that they don't engage in team learning behaviors. Two studies indeed showed that high time pressure in negotiation results in less integrative agreement and more fixed pie perceptions, which means that people stick with their own ideas and don't integrate ideas of others [54].

RESEARCH ON TIME PRESSURE, TASK COMPLEXITY AND TEAMS

Akkermans [51] conducted a study using the business simulator described above [39,40]. Her research sample consisted of 99 teams (consisting of two people). Participants were first-year business economics students. Teams represented the management of different companies and were required to make decisions. All companies playing the game were linked with each other through a computer network. The development of the markets was, for the main part, determined by all the teams together (the cumulative decisions of all the teams represent market dynamics). The business environment consisted of four markets: a market for consumption goods, a labor market, a market for investments and a credit market. There were five types of actors in this simulation: companies, consumers, employees, banks and governments. The computer model simulated the decisions of the consumers, employees, banks and government. The teams made decisions about their own company in which five decision variables were important: their price, the wage, the labor demand and the purchase of machines, machines newly ordered and the type of newly ordered machines. The simulator gave the teams the opportunity to change their policy every month (sixty seconds represent the time of one month). Every sixty seconds, teams had to make decisions about the decision variables. Their goal was to maximize the value of their companies by the end of the game. This value consisted of Market share, Sales and Equity Capital.

Perceived Task Complexity and Perceived Time Pressure were measured with a questionnaire containing validated scales taken from published research [55]. The items measuring perceived task difficulty were: 'I would characterize the game as (1=easy/7=difficult)', 'I would characterize the game as (1=challenging/7=difficult)' and 'I would characterize the task as 1=effortless / 7=demanding). The items measuring perceived time pressure were: 'More time would have helped us to achieve a better result in this management game (1=strongly disagree/7=strongly agree), 'In this game we had enough time to decide what we were going to do (1=strongly disagree/7=strongly agree)' and 'In terms of our performance, time was not a critical factor (1=strongly disagree/7=strongly agree).

Team learning behaviors were measured with validated scales measuring three aspects of the team learning behavior: construction, co-construction and constructive conflict [37] Examples of items measuring these team learning behaviors were respectively: 'In this team, we listened carefully to each other', 'Information of team members was complemented with information of other team members' and 'We tended to handle differences in opinion directly'. The answers on these questions could range from 1= I disagree completely to 7= I agree completely.

For measurement of teams' *Shared Mental Models* we build an expert model first. The developer of the simulator was asked to serve as player in the simulator and asked to think aloud about the five decision variables mentioned earlier [39,40]. This think-aloud protocol was analyzed by looking at the concepts used (content) when making decisions. Many concepts appeared to play a role in making these decisions and different concepts played a role in different decision variables for example when he had to make a decision about the price of the product of his company, he used different concepts to make this decision than when he had to make a decision about the investments of his company. Examples of concepts are: sales, competitor's price, production capacity, consumer demand etc. Finally, we build decision matrices consisting of decisions variables in the simulator and business concepts underlying these decisions. The expert was again asked to fill out this matrix and indicate for each of the mentioned decision variables which concepts were important in making a decision about the decision variable (structure). This was done to check whether the same concepts were mentioned in this matrix as were mentioned in the think-aloud protocol and this was the case.

The final version of the matrix was used to assess the shared mental models of the student teams. At the end of the simulation, students were asked to fill out the matrix and indicate for each of the mentioned decision variables which concepts were, according to them, important in making a decision about these decision variables by marking the appropriate cell(s). Based on these cognitive maps of individual mental models, the shared mental model of the team was computed.

RESULTS AND DISCUSSION

Table 1 contains the correlations between the variables measured in Akkerman's [51] study. She found a positive correlation between Perceived Time Pressure and Perceived Task Complexity. Next, it was found that teams who perceive a higher task complexity perceive that their team performance is poorer. Despite the lack of correlations between Team Learning Behavior and Time Pressure and Task Complexity, it was found that Team Learning Behavior is indeed related to Team Performance. This finding is consistent with the Van den Bossche studies [38].

Contrary to our expectations we found no significant main effects for Team Time Pressure and Team Task Complexity on Team Learning Behaviors, and there was no significant interaction between Team Time Pressure and Team Task Complexity. Although previous research has demonstrated that higher team learning behaviors in the interaction of the team lead to higher sharedness of the mental model, our outcomes did not support this. Regression analysis showed a non-significant positive regression coefficient between team learning behaviors and sharedness.

Table 1. Means, standard deviations and Intercorrelations (N=99 teams)

Variables	Mean	SD	1	2	3	4	5	6	7
(1) Time Pressure	3.80	1.2	-						
(2) Task Complexity	4.79	.9	**.48**	-					
(3) Team Learning Behavior	5.81	.6	.04	.01	-				
(4) Team Performance	5.64	.9	-.15	**-.20**	**.55**	-			
(5) Sharedness	28.04	11.5	.16	-.11	.14	.01	-		
(6) Market Share	50.00	28.7	-.07	-.07	-.14	-.01	.07	-	
(7) Sales	50.00	28.7	.02	-.13	-.11	.14	.17	**.40**	-
(8) Equity	50.00	28.7	**-.30**	**-.21**	.06	**.34**	-.04	.05	.07

Note. Correlations greater than (-).20 are significant at the .05 level. Significant correlations are printed in **bold**.

A possible explanation for the non-significant results of Time Pressure and Task Complexity on Team Learning Behaviors and the subsequent non significant results of Team Learning Behaviors on Sharedness may be that team learning behaviors do not play a mediating role in the effects of Time Pressure and Task Complexity on Sharedness. A second possible explanation may be that team members did not want to fall short to their partner/ team member with which they worked for two weeks when filling out the questionnaires. It may be possible that items on team learning behaviors elicited socially desirable answers and this could also be an explanation of the non significant results found in this study.

Detailed regression analyses demonstrated that Time Pressure and Task Complexity had a significant direct effect on sharedness [51]. When partialling out the correlation between Time Pressure and Task Complexity we found significant effects. Time Pressure had a positive effect on Sharedness, while team Task Complexity had a significant negative effect on both. These findings indicate that when Time Pressure is high, the team members can use each other's knowledge to perform well, but when Task Complexity is high, both team members don't have the knowledge and skills to help each other to successfully perform the task. This finding confirms previous research on the effects of Time Pressure and Task Complexity on Team Performance [38]. Akkermans' [51] research demonstrated as well that Time Pressure and Task Complexity had negative effects on one of the objective outcome variables: Equity.

At first sight, no relation was established between shared mental models and team performance indicators. However, further analyses revealed that if also the quality of the content of the mental models was taken into consideration, a relation is established between shared mental models and performance [51]. This is concurrent with recent insights in the shared mental model literature [38].

In general it can be said that this research provides indications that teams may suffer more when Task Complexity is perceived as high as compared to perceived Time Pressure. Akkermans emphasized that Time Pressure can be manageable for teams (through improved coordination and communication), while Complexity serves as a cognitive constraint. It is a more viable option for teams to change working procedures between team members, than aiming for the virtually impossible: acquiring necessary knowledge and skills while working on the task.

The latter finding brings us back to the potentials of Crew Resource Management (CRM) for teams that encounter complex problem situations under time pressure. We argued in the introduction of this article that CRM has proven to be beneficial for aviation. The present findings of Akkermans' work points out in similar directions for business. Of course, more can and needs to be done to improve our measures and research methods, but by following the leads from CRM it may be possible to improve our research and methods for team training in business.

CONCLUSION

The research conducted in our department on Team Learning Behaviors is an attempt to capture essential team processes, and provide improved insights on how social processes within teams determine cognitive performance. The present article presents an overview of our research program and how its findings can be used to interpret team work, and improve team training. While our research is in progress, we hope that we can make a contribution to team work in business. But we do feel that this work can contribute to the acceleration of research in health care to improve patient safety through improved team work. From that perspective, it is interesting to note that leading researchers in this field – Edmondson and her co-workers – are researchers working at a prominent business school, but who were capable to apply theories and conceptual frameworks about team learning in the field of health care [6,7,8].

In our view the field of medicine can gain substantially from insights on team-work and communication collected in different fields such as aviation or business. Our research provides strong evidence that team member's belief about their team have a substantial impact on team learning and team performance. For example, we found that psychological safety is a variable that has a very strong effect on team learning and the development of shared mental models. This confirms Edmondson's [6] earlier research on reporting errors in nursing teams and the way this is related to teams' perceptions of psychological safety.

We recommend that the field of medicine must establish more attention to team processes with input from research on CRM in aviation, and team processes in business. In our view the field of medicine has become too complex to attribute errors to individuals, adhering to a blame and shame culture. By following the examples set in other complex domains, it should be possible to find a balance between the individual professional autonomy on one hand, and the responsibilities of individual health care workers at an aggregated level: teams, departments, or even the hospital as organization. As in aviation, safety is not only the individual's responsibility. It requires more. Even although we may see many opportunities to share our insights, or implement them in organization practice, it requires that health care professionals are willing to adapt our insights and modify them for their own professional context.

REFERENCES

[1]   Cohen SG, Bailey DE. What makes teams work: Group effectiveness research from the shop floor to the executive suite. Journal of Management 1997;23:239-290.

[2]   Salas E, Sims DE, Burke CS. Is there a "Big Five" in teamwork? Small Group Research 2005;36:555-599.

[3]   Beers PJ. Negotiating common ground: Tools for multidisciplinary teams. Unpublished doctoral dissertation. Heerlen: Open Universiteit Nederland; 2005.

[4]   Vennix JAM. Group model building. Facilitating team learning using system dynamics. Chichester: Hohn Wiley & Sons; 1996.

[5]   Hackman JR, editor. Groups that work (and those that don't). Creating conditions for effective teamwork. San Francisco, CA: Jossey-Bass; 1989.

[6]   Edmondson AC. Psychological safety and learning behavior in work teams. Administrative Science Quarterly 1999:44;350-383.

[7]   Edmondson AC, Bohmer RM, Pisano, GP. Disrupted Routines: Team Learning and New Technology Implementation in Hospitals. Administrative Science Quarterly 2001:46;685-716.

[8]   Edmondson AC. Speaking Up in the Operating Room: How Team Leaders Promote Learning in Interdisciplinary Action Teams. Journal of Management Studies 2003:40;1419-1452.

[9]   Lingard L, Espin S, Whyte S, Regehr G, Baker GR, Reznick R, Bohnen J, Orser B, Doran D, Grober E. Communication failures in the operating room: an observational classification of recurrent types and effects. Qual. Saf. Health Care 2004:13;330-334.

[10]   Davies JM. Medical Applications of Crew Resource Management. In Salas E, Bowers CA, Edens E. editors. Improving Teamwork in Organizations. Applications of Resource Management Training. Lawrence Erlbaum. Mahwah, NY; 2001:265-282.

[11]   Salas E, Bowers CA, Edens E. Improving Teamwork in Organizations. Applications of Resource Management Training. Mahwah, NY: Lawrence Erlbaum; 2001.

[12]   Kline DA. (2005). Intuitive team decision making. In Montgomery H, Lipshitz R, Brehmer B, editors. How Professionals Make Decisions. Mahwah, NJ: Lawrence Erlbaum Associates; 2005:171-182.

[13]   Barron B. Achieving coordination in collaborative problem-solving groups. The Journal of the Learning Sciences 2000: 9;403-436.

[14]   Barron B. When smart groups fail. The Journal of the Learning Sciences 2003:12;307-359.

[15]   Knight D, Pearce CL, Smith KG, Olian JD, Sims HP, Smith KA, Flood P. Top management team diversity, group process, and strategic consensus. Strategic Management Journal 1999:20;445 – 465.

[16]   Ericsson KA, Smith J, editors. Toward a General Theory of Expertise; Prospects and Limits. Cambridge, MA: Cambridge University Press; 1993.

[17]   Patel VL, Arocha JF, Kaufman DR, editors. Expertise and Tacit Knowledge in Medicine. In Sternberg R, Horvath J. Tacit Knowledge in Professional Practice. Researcher and Practioner Perspectives. LEA Mahwah, NJ; 1999:75-99.

[18]   Schmidt HG, Boshuizen HPA. On the origin of intermediate effects in clinical case recall. Memory and Cognition 1993:21;338-351.

[19] Sternberg RJ, editor. The Nature of Cognition. Cambridge; MA: MIT Press; 1999.

[20] Wong, S. Collective cognition in team: The role of interactive learning and effects on team performance. Paper presented at the Academy of Management, Seattle; 2003.

[21] Roschelle J. Learning by collaborating: Convergent conceptual change. Journal of the Learning Sciences 1992:2;235-276.

[22] Langfield-Smith K. Exploring the need for a shared cognitive map. Journal of Management Studies 1992:29;349-368.

[23] Marks MA, Mathieu JE, Zaccaro SJ. A temporally based framework and taxonomy of team processes. Academy of Management Review 2001:26;356-376.

[24] Cannon-Bowers JA, Salas E. Reflections on shared cognition. Journal of Organizational Behavior 2001:22;195-202.

[25] Nosek JT, McNeese MD. Issues for knowledge management from experiences in supporting group knowledge elicitation & creation in ill-defined, emerging situations. Paper presented at the AAAI Spring Symposium Artificial intelligence in knowledge Management, Stanford University; 1997.

[26] De Dreu CKW, Weingart LR. Task versus relationship conflict, team performance, and team member satisfaction: A meta-analysis. Journal of Applied Psychology 2003:88:741-749.

[27] Klimoski R, Mohammed, S. Team mental model: Construct or metaphor? Journal of Management 1994:20;403-437.

[28] Baker MJ. Negotiation in collaborative problem-solving dialogues. In Beun RJ, Baker M, Reiner M editors. Dialogue and instruction. Modeling interaction in intelligent tutoring systems. Berlin: Springer-Verlag; 1995;39-55.

[29] Alpay L, Giboin A, Dieng R. Accidentology: An example of problem solving by multiple agents with multiple representations. In van Someren MW, Reimann P, Boshuizen HPA, de Jong T editors. Learning with multiple representations. Amsterdam: Pergamon; 1998;152-174.

[30] Baker M. A model for negotiation in teaching-learning dialogues. Journal of Artificial Intelligence in Education 1994:5;199-254.

[31] Arrow H, McGrath JE, Berdahl JL. Small Groups as complex systems. Formation, coordination, development and adaptation. Sage Publications, Inc: Thousand Oaks, California; 2000.

[32] Mullen B, Copper C. The relation between group cohesiveness and performance: An integration. Psychological Bulletin 1994:115;210-227.

[33] Van der Vegt G, Emans B, van de Vliert E. Motivating effects of task and outcome interdepence in work teams. Group & Organization Management 1998:23;124-143.

[34] Wageman, R. Interdependence and group effectiveness. Administrative Science Quarterly 1995:40;145-180.

[35] Shea GP, Guzzo RA. Groups as human resources. In Rowland KM, Ferris GR, editors. Research in personnel and human resources management. Greenwich, CT: JAI Press; 1987:323-356.

[36] Lomi A, Larsen ER, Ginsberg A. Adaptive learning in organizations: A system-dynamics-based exploration. Journal of Management 1997:23;561-582.

[37] Van den Bossche P, Gijselaers WH, Segers MSR, Kirschner PA. Social and Cognitive factors driving teamwork in collaborative learning environments: Team learning beliefs and behaviors. Small Group Research, 2006:37;490-521.

[38] Van den Bossche P. Minds in Teams. The influence of social and cognitive factors on team learning. Unpublished Doctoral Thesis. Maastricht: Maastricht University; 2006.

[39] Woltjer, G. Coordination in a Macroeconomic Game. Its design and its role in education and experiments. Maastricht: Universitaire Pers Maastricht; 1995.

[40] Woltjer, G. Decisions and Macro-economics: Development and Implementation of a simulation game. Journal of Economic Education 2005:36.

[41] Jehn KA. (1995). A multimethod examination of the benefits and detriments of intragroup conflict. Administrative Science Quarterly 1995:40;256-282.

[42] Williams KY, O'Reilly CA. Demography and diversity in organizations: A review of 40 years of research. Research in Organizational Behavior 1998:20;77-140.

[43] Pelled LH, Eisenhardt KM, Xin KR. Exploring the black box: An analysis of work group diversity, conflict, and performance. Administrative Science Quarterly 1999:44;1-28.

[44] West MA, Hirst G, Richter A, Shipton H. Twelve steps to heaven: Succesfully managing change through developing innovative teams. European Journal of Work and Organizational Psychology 2004:13;269-299.

[45] Van den Bossche P, Gijselaers WH, Segers, M, Woltjer, G. Sharing expertise in management: An experimental study on team learning and its effect on shared mental models. Paper presented at the Academy of Management, Hawaii; 2005.

[46] Keyton J. The relational side of groups. Small Group Research 2000:31;387-396.

[47] De Dreu CKW, Weingart LR. Task versus relationship conflict, team performance, and team member satisfaction: A meta-analysis. Journal of Applied Psychology 2003:88;741-749.

[48] Bantel K, Jackson S. Top management and innovations in banking: Does the composition of the top team make a difference? Strategic Management Journal, Summer Special Issue 1989:10;107-124.

[49] Bantel, K. Top Team, Environment, and Performance Effects on Strategic Planning Formality. Group & Organization Management 1993:18;436-458.

[50] Hackman, J.R. (1987). The design of work teams. In Handbook of Organizational Behavior, 315-342. Englewood Cliffs, NJ: Prentice Hall.

[51] Akkermans M. Team Mental Modelling. The effects of task complexity and time pressure on the development and quality of shared mental models. Unpublished Master Thesis. Maastricht: Maastricht University; 2006.

[52] Baumann MR, Bonner BL, Reeshad S. The effects of member expertise on group decision-making and performance. Organizational Behavior and Human Decision Processes 2002:88;719-736.

[53] Kruglanski AW. The psychology of being 'right': The problem of accuracy in social perception and cognition, Psychological Bulletin 1989:106;395-409.

[54] De Dreu C. Time pressure and the closing of the mind in negotiation. Organizational Behavior and Human Decision Processes 2003:91;280-295.

[55] Topi H,. Valacich JS. Hoffer JA The effects of task complexity and time availability limitations on human performance in database query tasks. International Journal of Human-Computer Studies 2005:62;349-379.

In: Dresden Teamwork Concept for Medical…
Editor: Axel R. Heller

ISBN 978-1-60692-307-8
© 2009 Nova Science Publishers, Inc.

Chapter 5

Team Management in Helicopter Emergency Medical Services (HEMS)

Michael P. Müller, Mike Hänsel and Axel R. Heller

Department of Anesthesiology & Critical Care Medicine,
University Hospital Carl Gustav Carus, University of Technology, Dresden, Germany

Abstract

In Germany Helicopter Emergency Medical Service (HEMS) teams consist of one pilot, one emergency physician, and one paramedic being additionally trained in aviation procedures. HEMS are assigned to the most complex situations, even when ground EMS are already on site. The crew members in distinct situations may well indentify individually different priorities regarding the objectives of the mission. Thus, a shared mental model of the team is the key success factor for effective and safe patient treatment.

In a variety of examples tasks of the team members and goals of the entire rescue mission are analyzed, being characterized by a dynamic high risk environment, the multidisciplinarity of the team as well as time- and emotional pressure. Since one rescue mission may be divided into different episodes leadership and followership roles change depending on the progression of the mission underscoring the impact of good team performance and shared mental models. From this point of view training of non technical skills in medicine is, thus, indispensable. To achieve good Crew Resource Management (CRM) the Dresden Six Step Approach of CRM is described improving team performance by introducing psychological know how into CRM focusing on shared mental models and team effectiveness.

HEMS in Germany

In 1970 the first rescue helicopter was put into service in Germany. This service aimed at early medical care for traumatized patients especially on the motorways as well as fast transport to the trauma centers. By this time an ambulance system had already been established in Germany involving physicians on the scene of accidents. During the following decades ambulances and helicopters had increasing numbers of rescue missions not only due to increasing traffic but mainly because physician staffed ambulances and helicopters were now additionally posted to rescue missions with non-traumatized but seriously ill patients such as cardiac arrests, or dyspnoea. Meanwhile over 50 rescue helicopters are in service and available for rescue missions from 7 a.m. to sunset covering a radius of 50 km each. After alert is given the rescue helicopter takes off within 2 minutes and usually reaches its destination in less than 15 minutes. In Germany air rescue bases on average have more than 1,000 missions per year. Main restriction for the HEMS system are non- visual flight conditions such as night time and bad weather conditions, not allowing rescue missions. Additional helicopters are in service for inter-hospital transfer of critically ill patients. These helicopters usually run 24 hours and are mostly manned with two pilots during night times.

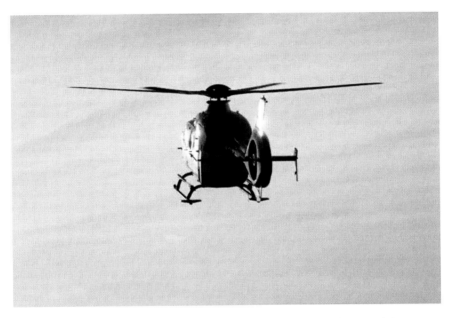

Figure 1. Christoph 38 Rescue helicopter, German Air Rescue, Dresden (Photograph by courtesy of Daniel Becker).

TEAM MEMBERS IN HEMS MISSIONS

Most rescue helicopters in Germany are staffed with one pilot, one paramedic, and one physician. Some helicopters are available for mountain rescue missions and are equipped with a cable winch and are manned with a flight technician for winch operations.

Pilot: One characteristic of the pilot's job is that the helicopter has to be airborne within two minutes after alarm. Furthermore minimization of the time from alert until reaching the destination may decide about the patient's life or death putting stress and emotional pressure on the pilot. The scene of the emergency has to be found from the helicopter and a suitable landing place without obstacles such as power lines has to be identified. Sometimes a rescue mission has to be abandoned due to deteriorated weather conditions.

Paramedic: The paramedic has to complete a one week course for HEMS crew members (HCM) containing teaching modules on weather, navigation, radio, and technical aspects of helicopters. Furthermore, the paramedic has to complete 10 rescue missions under supervision. Further restrictions such as a minimum of rescue missions to be completed as a HCM per year may apply according to the organization's operating manual.

Physician: In Germany specialization as pre-hospital emergency physician requires a minimum of two years experience in anesthesiology, surgery or neurosurgery, neurology, general medicine, or pediatrics. Furthermore, a two week course on emergency medicine has to be completed and the respective physician has to work for at least six months in anesthesiology, on an intensive care unit or in an emergency department. There is no special training for air rescue except for safety instructions regarding the helicopter.

COMMON MISSION GOALS AND CONFLICTS OF INTEREST

As already might be concluded from their individual training during helicopter rescue missions the crew members sometimes may well indentify individually distinct priorities regarding the objectives of the mission. The following example may serve to facilitate understanding of the different perception and aims.

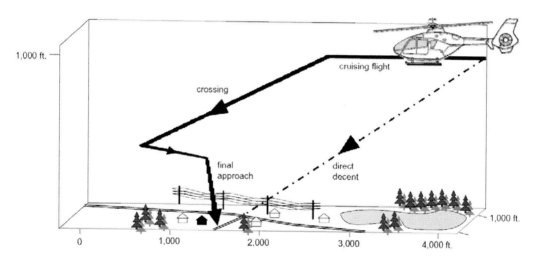

Figure 2. Approach of helicopter in a rescue mission. Standard procedure with crossing potential landing zone (black house) and final approach in a triangular course.

The rescue operations control centre received a call from a woman reporting on her husband (53 years old) suddenly having been fallen unconscious and looking cyanotic. An ambulance has been assigned but will need approximately 20 minutes to reach the patient. The dispatcher orders the rescue helicopter to the case which could reach the patient in less than 10 minutes. Six minutes after being alerted the patients' house is in sight of the helicopter crew (Figure 2, black house). Standard procedure for the pilot is to cross the location to identify the optimal place for landing and do the final approach in a triangular course. The emergency physician, however, asks the pilot for a direct decent of the helicopter without any delay because the patient is supposed to have a cardiac arrest. In case of a cardiac arrest even short delays of beginning the cardiopulmonary resuscitation may result in severe neurological sequel. After landing on the street the paramedic secures the helicopter to prevent a motor vehicle accident.

Which goals have the three team members in that mission? Let us put oneself in the *pilot's* place. His job is to fly the helicopter and bring the medical team and the patient safely to the destination. In the previously described situation a safe landing procedure after crossing the scene of the emergency causes a delay. While crossing the landing area the pilot can identify potential obstacles and hazards. Reports from previous rescue helicopter accidents clearly show that this procedure is important for maximum safety in rescue missions [1]. For this reason the pilot accepts the delay.

The *physician* aims to reach the patient as soon as possible. Especially young physicians without experience in air rescue may not understand competing interests in special scenarios. In our scenario the physician puts pressure onto the pilot when asking him to land without delay. It has to be questioned which information the pilot needs about the medical condition of the patient as stress may cause errors or unsafe actions.

In the present case the *paramedic* secures the helicopter after landing lastly causing delay in patient care since he shows up at the scene of the emergency (house approximately 200 m from the landing place) some minutes later as the physician. In fact the patient was pulseless with the need for cardiopulmonary resuscitation. As there were no further personnel, the physician had to commence alone. The paramedic in his double role as HCM has to assist the pilot regarding aeronautical aspects and to assist the physician regarding medical treatment and therefore may be confronted with a conflict of interests.

How relevant is a potential conflict of interest in the helicopter team regarding the safety of the mission? Scrutinizing the safety in HEMS missions in Germany Hinkelbein and colleagues studied accidents in rescue helicopter missions in Germany and found 24 crashes in a five-years period representing an accident rate of 0.54 per 10,000 missions [1;2]. Fifty-four percent of the accidents happened during final approach or landing. This flight section is quite dangerous and the team should support the pilot in looking out for safe landing places and not putting pressure on him.

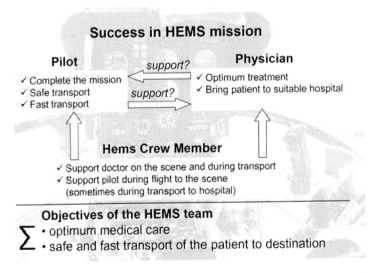

Figure 3. Objectives of individuals in rescue helicopter teams and objectives of the complete team.

The effect of emotional pressure on the crew members during a rescue mission with its potential risks is shown in the following example. A rescue mission is assigned in the afternoon of a misty winter day. Although the weather conditions are poor, the pilot decides to fly the mission after a short briefing with his team and with weather services. Shortly before reaching the destination he again discusses the conditions with his team and asks the HCM to inform the rescue operations control center that they possibly would have to abandon the mission due to deteriorating weather. Operations command in reply recommended to go ahead because a young child is seriously injured. The helicopter reached the scene of the accident and the child had only minor injuries. One could question whether the pilot should get this unverified information. On one hand he would take the importance of a mission into account when balancing risk and benefit, on the other hand this information puts him under pressure. From the physician's point of view the mission was not that important. He knew that the scene of the accident is only 10 kilometers away from the next trauma centre and that there are physician staffed ambulances (which would reach the scene less than 10 minutes later than the helicopter). He told the pilot that it would probably not have a great impact on the patients´ outcome if they would have cancelled their mission.

Not few missions are abandoned due to bad weather conditions. In preparation of transfer flights between hospitals, in particular the weather conditions have to meet minimum standards being defined by the respective organization. In theory the regulations are clear and one can hardly believe that problems may arise. However, when weather conditions are slightly worse than minimum standards the pilot may decide to fly the mission. In the sense of good Crew Resource Management (CRM) success of a mission can be assessed in Figure 3.

The pilot may feel being put under emotional pressure to perform a flight when conditions are too poor for a rescue mission. The physician may just await the pilot's decision and do a good job providing optimum medical treatment. However, in a good team he can support the pilot in the pre-flight briefing.

Here is an example for a HEMS team decision. The team of a rescue helicopter is alarmed for an urgent transfer of a patient from a general hospital in the area of Dresden to the university hospital. The patient has had an acute myocardial infarction and needs a coronary intervention which cannot be accomplished in this level 1 hospital. The time from the onset of the myocardial infarction to the intervention is outcome-relevant. The distance between the two hospitals is approximately 12 kilometers (road distance). The weather conditions have worsened during the last 30 minutes and the visibility just meets the minimum requirements. Immediately after being alarmed the pilot calls weather forecast service and gets the information that there won't be better conditions but perhaps thunderstorms in the region during the next two hours. The pilot decides that the mission could be done. Meanwhile the physician via phone interchanges information on the patient with his colleague in charge in the peripheral hospital (as it is usually done prior to a transfer mission). The patient is in a critical state and the physician ordered helicopter transport believing that this would take less time than ground transport with the ambulance.

In a pre-flight briefing the pilot states that the weather conditions are satisfactory at the moment but may well worsen which would force the pilot to cancel the mission. Cancellation of the mission in flight would additionally prolong definite ground transportation of the patient. The physician shares his thoughts and concerns about the patient with the crew stating that severe arrhythmias requiring cardiopulmonary resuscitation may occur during the flight to the university hospital. This information is of great value for the pilot as cardiopulmonary resuscitation in the passenger cabin is difficult to perform and the physician would need the assistance by the paramedic/ HCM in this case. In bad weather conditions the paramedic is, likewise, a valuable resource in the cockpit as he helps navigating and watches out for traffic. After weighing threads and benefits of an airborne rescue mission for the patient, the team decides that ground transport is safer, because when cardiopulmonary resuscitation has to commence an ambulance car may easily stop [3]. Furthermore the time advantage of HEMS transportation may be neglected (only 12 kilometers to drive): A common problem is that the general hospitals often are in shortness of physicians on duty to accompany the patient during the ambulance transport. The helicopter always is staffed with a physician which is – among others – an argument for air transport. In bad weather conditions and when the patient is so critical that air transport may be associated with increased risk, all these aspects have to be taken into account.

The complete team should build a shared mental model (see also chapter 4) which includes a commitment to the common objectives during the mission (Figure 3). According to Cannon-Bowers and colleagues all team members need three knowledge components: knowledge of own capabilities (meta-knowledge), knowledge of the task(s), and knowledge about the capabilities of the other team members [4]. In the previously described case the team decided to reject the mission.

LEADERSHIP AND FOLLOWERSHIP IN RESCUE HELICOPTER MISSIONS

One interesting aspect in helicopter teams is that a mission can be divided into 3 sections: The flight to the scene of the emergency or accident, the treatment of the patient(s) on the scene, and the flight to the hospital. In the first phase the pilot is the team leader and the two other team members are supporting him according to their capabilities. In the second phase the physician leads the team as he is in charge for the medical treatment. Although the pilot does usually not have a medical education he commonly supports the medical crew in special situations. If for instance there is no ambulance at the scene and the medical crew has a high workload the pilot may perform specific tasks according to his experience and training. Chest compressions are an example for a skill which can be performed by the pilot which is very helpful for the medical crew in cardiac arrest scenarios. During the third phase there are shared responsibilities as the pilot is in charge for the helicopter and the physician is responsible for the medical treatment. It is essential that the team communicates effectively before and during the flight [5]. Some aspects of good teamwork are as follows: **Communication on different perspectives** and of the **plan** (and alternative plans) the team will follow. The physician mostly has the nearest hospital in mind which will provide optimal care for the patient. The team has to discuss whether this hospital can be reached (weather conditions, fuel) or the hospital actually has the resources to take over and treat the patient (operating room capacities, capacities on intensive care unit etc.). Sometimes an alternative destination should be defined if it is not clear whether the conditions will change during the flight (weather, patient's state).

Early communication of concerns and important information. If the weather conditions worsen during the flight the pilot should share these information with the team early enough. The crew should be able to think about alternative destinations (if not already done prior to the flight) without high time pressure. On the other side the physician, likewise, has to share aviation relevant medical information with he team. If he expects a critical arrhythmia in a patient probably requiring electric cardioversion or defibrillation he has to announce that. Defibrillation may cause electric interference with instruments in the cockpit. Due to engine noise crew communication near and within the helicopter is much more difficult than in ground EMS. Therefore, during the flight the crew members exchange information via intercom. Moreover, the pilot and the physician have no eye contact.

Give and receive feedback. Because of the different professions the members of the helicopter team may sometimes not understand their teammates' actions and plans. To avoid emotional conflicts a debriefing is valuable. If the pilot has to abort a mission the debriefing may establish understanding for his behaviour. If new pilots commence their job in air rescue, feedback from the physician's point of view may be helpful after a mission to improve understanding for the medical part and to reduce emotional pressure.

Being a good leader and a good follower. Due to the changing leadership role during a rescue mission, the team members have changing duties. In one phase of the mission they may have to lead the team whereas in another phase they work as a follower.

DRESDEN CREW RESOURCE MANAGEMENT TRAINING CONCEPT

It has been recognized more than 30 years ago that human errors contribute to 50-80% of incidents in aviation.

According to regulations by the Joint Aviation Authorities (JAA) the flight crew has to be trained in crew resource management, which means the application of the principles of human factors. Regrettably the physician is regarded as "medical passenger" and not as a crew member. Thus, most physicians working in German rescue helicopter services are not trained in CRM. We therefore claim that CRM training is mandatory for the entire HEMS crew (in aviation even cabin crew members have to take part in CRM training). CRM seminars focus on improvement of training strategies, team relationship, and staff and resource management. Pizzi et al. conclude that the use of CRM, as has been in use for many years in aviation, has tremendous potential [6].

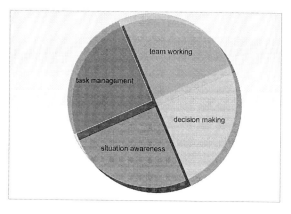

Figure 4. Categories of CRM training.

In the Dresden interdisciplinary medical simulation center ISIMED (www.isimed.info) we established a non-technical skills course concept, called "six step approach", which combines the two strategies of CRM training and patient simulation [7;8]. The course was developed by physicians and psychologists and consists of four main modules according to the four main categories (Figure 4) of the anesthetists' non-technical skills found by Flin et al. [9]. Module one "situation awareness" is focused on mediating skills in developing and maintaining awareness of a situation based on perceiving environmental elements. The second module "task management" targets management of actual resources and organization of tasks to achieve goals. In module three "teamwork" takes the developing skills for working in a group environment center. The fourth module "decision-making" deals with decisions or judgments/diagnoses about a situation. Each module is scheduled for 90 min. For us it was important that the course design facilitates adopting error management strategies which would be available in various (realistic) situations. Therefore we developed the following six steps training approach combining psychological exercises on error management with practical patient simulation (Figure 5). This course design is used in each of the four non-technical skill modules:

Step 1: Medical instructors demonstrate a short simulation scenario practicing good CRM behavior. Participants are asked to discuss the key elements of CRM in relation to the demonstrated scenario. This exercise lasts around 25 min and defines the course objectives. In this step good CRM behavior is conveyed by "model learning".

Step 2: During a 10-min lecture a psychological instructor teaches theories of human factors for the particular non-technical skill. Additionally examples for psychological effects with impact on the participants' daily work are demonstrated to point out human factor-associated problems.

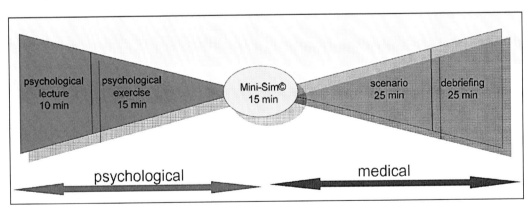

Figure 5. Six-Step approach in each unit. After presentation of good CRM performance by the instructors in a scenario (step 1) the further five steps are accomplished as depicted.

Step 3: Participants take part in exercises focusing on the psychological intention of the respective module. The participants deal with psychological content in the context of a realistic situation, therefore leading to a learning experience.

Step 4: During a 15 min exercise on a patient simulator participants have to apply the learned psychological strategy in step 3 to solve a medical problem. The fourth step is used as interface between the imparted knowledge of psychological strategies and the problems in the daily work environment, that's why it called "MiniSim".

Step 5: This step leads participants into a realistic emergency scenario. A team of three to four participants have to solve a critical medical incident on their own. With one or two intermediate-fidelity patient simulators, pre-hospital emergencies as well as emergencies in a casualty department are simulated. During this step, the other participants are seated in a neighboring room and observe the scenario via a video display. These observers are asked to focus on the participants' implementation of the strategies learned previously.

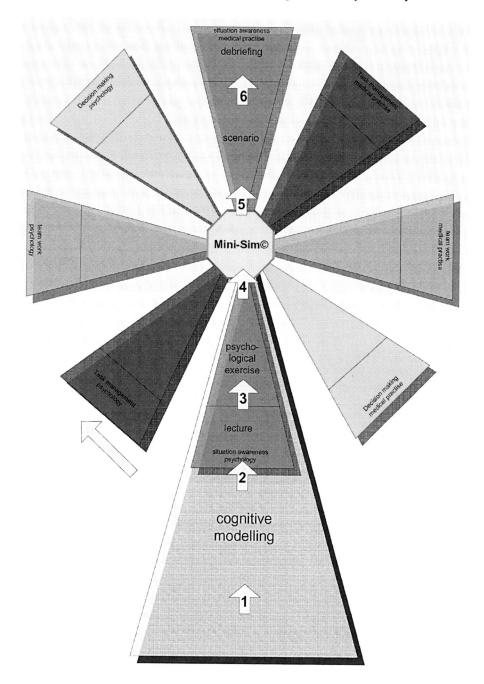

Figure 6. Dresden Six Step approach within the categories of teamwork. [8].

Step 6: The final step of each of the four modules is a debriefing after the scenario of step 5. A physician and the psychological instructor ask the active participants (hot seats) to estimate their technical and non-technical performance during the scenario with focus on the current module. Afterwards other participants discuss the team's actions by analyzing video sequences. In conclusion, participants are requested to name situations in their own working environment in which the non-technical skill demonstrated is essential and the acquired knowledge could be supportive. As depicted in Figure 6 as a wind wheel repetition of the six steps solidifies the trained CRM categories.

Evaluation results (of anesthetists and intensivists) of the six step approach has shown that a stepwise approximation from teaching theoretical CRM strategies to solving realistic emergency scenarios can support transfer of good CRM behavior in the daily work environment.

CONCLUSION

In Germany, Helicopter Emergency Medical Services (HEMS) represent the highest level of emergency treatment know how. HEMS are thus assigned to the most complex situations, even when ground EMS are already on site. Team Management tasks in HEMS are characterized by a dynamic high risk environment, the multidisciplinarity of the team as well as time- and emotional pressure. Dynamic decision making and Crew resource Management are key skills in aviation. Transferring this experience to medicine, in particular to emergency cases increases efficacy of patient care and at the same time controls risks.

During the HEMS rescue mission goals of the team dynamically have to be adapted to current needs (medical, aviation, tactical). Because of the multitude of information to be processed and communicated across professional boundaries good leadership and good followership in dynamically changing roles is vital for HEMS team success.

Training of non technical skills is, thus, indispensable. The Dresden Six Step Approach of Crew Resource Management improves Team performance by introducing psychological know how into CRM focusing on shared mental models and team effectiveness

REFERENCES

[1] Hinkelbein J, Dambier M, Viergutz T, Genzwurker H. A 6-year analysis of German emergency medical services helicopter crashes. J Trauma 2008 Jan;64(1):204-10.

[2] Dambier M, Hinkelbein J. Analysis of 2004 German general aviation aircraft accidents according to the HFACS model. Air Med J 2006 Nov;25(6):265-9.

[3] Heller AR, Muller MP, Frank MD, Dressler J. [Rigor mortis -- a definite sign of death?]. Anasthesiol Intensivmed Notfallmed Schmerzther 2005 Apr;40(4):225-9.

[4] Cannon-Bowers JA, Salas E, Converse S. Shared mental models in expert team decision making. In: Castellan Jr JN, editor. Individual and group decision making.Hillsdale NJ: Lawrence Erlbaum; 1993. p. 221-46.

[5]   Muller M, Bergmann B, Koch T, Heller A. [Dynamic decision making in emergency medicine. Example of paraplegia after a traffic accident]. Anaesthesist 2005 Aug;54(8):781-6.

[6]   Pizzi L, Goldfarb NI, Nash DB. Crew resource management and its applications in medicine. Making Health Care Safer: A Critical Analysis of Patient Safety Practices. 43 ed. Rockville: Agency for Healthcare Research and Quality; 2001. p. 501-10.

[7]   Mueller MP, Heller AR, Koch T. A new simulator-based psychological training on crisis management. Med Educ 2005 Nov;39(11):1155.

[8]   Muller MP, Hansel M, Stehr SN, Fichtner A, Weber S, Hardt F, et al. Six steps from head to hand: a simulator based transfer oriented psychological training to improve patient safety. Resuscitation 2007 Apr;73(1):137-43.

[9]   Flin R, Maran N. Identifying and training non-technical skills for teams in acute medicine. Qual Saf Health Care 2004 Oct;13 Suppl 1:i80-4.:i80-i84.

In: Dresden Teamwork Concept for Medical...
Editor: Axel R. Heller

ISBN 978-1-60692-307-8
© 2009 Nova Science Publishers, Inc.

Chapter 6

IMPLEMENTATION OF A CRITICAL INCIDENT REPORTING SYSTEM INTO HEALTHCARE HIGH RISK ORGANIZATIONS

Matthias Hübler and Angela K. Möllemann

Department of Anesthesiology and Intensive Care, University Hospital Carl Gustav Carus, Technical University Dresden, Germany

ABSTRACT

In 1999, the report "To Err is Human: building a safer health care system" was published by the American Institute of Medicine. This report and many publications thereafter confronted us with growing evidence that healthcare systems are not as safe as they could be. It is now well accepted that our medical services - unintentionally - sometimes not only fail to improve patients but also cause avoidable damage. In recognition of this, patient safety has become a fundamental part of the drive to improve quality into healthcare organizations.

One of the most frustrating aspects regarding patient safety is the apparent failure of health-care systems to learn from their mistakes. Too often health-care organizations ignore mishaps and hesitate to share information when an investigation has been carried out following an incident. As a consequence, the same mistakes occur repeatedly in many settings and patients continue to be harmed by preventable errors. Another drawback is that errors in complex work spaces such as hospitals are often not easily identified.

A primary aim to improve patient safety is to gather reliable information about flaws in the treatment course. This can be achieved using medical record review, analysis of adverse events, random screening, observational studies, and malpractice claims analysis or reporting systems. The article describes the aims and prerequisites to implement successfully an anonymous Critical Incident Reporting System into healthcare organizations. It further strengthens the importance of structured analysis of acquired data yielding measures to improve patient safety.

5.1 BENEFITS OF RISK MANAGEMENT IN HEALTHCARE ORGANIZATIONS

Industrial risk and quality management yields zero error during the process of value creation. Medical treatments of patients are characterized by numerous interactions of different medical and paramedical professionals. It lies in the nature of these interactions that human factors play an important role to promote, induce or aggravate errors. It is therefore not surprising that all known error reporting systems established in health care organizations strengthen human factors. In the medical setting, aiming at zero error during the treatment course appears overambitious and a more realistic - and more human - aim should be aiming at error reduction.

The term "risk" is not trademarked or exactly defined. Every interest group uses their own definition and therefore definitions differ among each group: Lawyers and third party insurers focus on different risks than hospital administrations. Press offices deal with other risks than kitchen facilities. Nurses and physicians think mostly about patients and their treatments when they are asked about risk in the hospital. Risk also implies for some people positive opportunities, e.g., risk-reward-ratio in the stock market. It is therefore evident, that risk perception depends on work environment, moral concepts and many personal factors.

Risk is mathematically defined as likelihood of a negative incidence whereas business economists expand this likelihood of a negative incidence by multiplying it with the financial impact. In the setting of risk management the term "risk" is usually defined as threats posed to values, circumstances or actions. **Risk management** acknowledges existing risks and focuses on:

- predicting the likelihood of errors,
- describing the impact of errors,
- ideally quantifying the impact of errors,
- analyzing errors,
- developing countermeasures, and
- implementing it.

Possible strategies of an effective risk management are therefore

- to avoid risks,
- to reduce risks (e.g., by reducing the likelihood of errors or their impact),
- to shift risks (e.g., towards third party insurers), and
- to bear the risks.

Risk management implies not only to detect errors in the process of value creation but also to realize the unique value of the detected errors to improve the process. If the gathered information is used progressively then risk management creates an atmosphere of confidence such that internal and external customers are convinced by the high quality and the safety of the processes. This stabilizes or even increases the number of customers (e.g., patients, referring physicians) although direct financial benefits of risk management in the medical setting are difficult to quantify.

The primary aim of a company or a hospital should be to manage detected or suspected risks and to avoid to be managed by them. Risks with monetary consequences are part of the mercantile risk management, whereas risks during the patients' treatment course with possible negative health effects belong to the medical risk management. It is obvious that both types of risk management overlap and that their mutual impacts depend on many factors such as patients' willingness for complaints and the number of claims for recourse initiated by health insurances. It is therefore not surprising that costs for liability insurances in the health sector increase and that hospitals with insufficient of absent risk management may even face difficulties getting insured.

5.2 CLINICAL RISK MANAGEMENT

The principal focuses of clinical risk management are to increase safety of patients and safety of medical staff. It is assumed that errors occur in the medical setting 10^5 times more often than in the industry. In the past, patients' mortality was perceived as the primary risk. Efforts during the last decades, such as improving education and equipments, decreased mortality rates tremendously. But also society changed at the same time and the absence of risks in daily life induced high individual demands regarding safety during treatment. As a consequence mortality data were replaced by morbidity data [3;12]. Today, not only treating physicians but also the public and individuals are sensitized regarding treatment side effects, treatment errors and mistreatments, which may lead to transitory or permanent health impairments and often cause personal or familiar grief.

Impressive improvements in medical treatments could not prevent that the number of detected treatment errors increases continuously. Although specific scientific data are missing it is a well accepted assumption that the relative frequency of treatment errors did not increase in the same degree over time. The higher rates of published treatment errors can be explained by the mentioned awareness rising, by the willingness of health workers to talk openly about errors, by the increase of specialized attorneys and finally by an increase in cases per time with shorter hospital stays. Following statements can be found in the report of the German government regarding medical treatment errors [6]:

- Suspected treatment errors are more often confirmed in small hospitals compared to big hospitals: In small hospitals with less than 200 beds 44 % of error reproaches were found to be true. The percentage values were 30 % in hospitals with 200 to 500 beds, 29 % in hospitals with more than 500 beds, and only 24 % in University hospitals, respectively.
- Physicians working in hospitals are approximately twice more often confronted with error reproaches than physicians working in private practice. The intense personal contact between physician and patient in private practice seems preventive compared to the anonymous atmosphere in hospitals, where time for personal interaction and communication is limited.
- In 20 % of acknowledged treatment errors, deficits in documentation were found to have either promoted the errors or to have led to a decision favoring the accusation.

- Insufficient patient information was at least a co-factor in 7 % of acknowledged treatment errors.
- Deficits in inter- and intradepartmental communication and coordination played an important role in 23 % of acknowledged treatment errors.

Teaching hospitals and University hospitals are threatened by additional factors with an impact on error rates [11]. These factors are:

- high percentage of trainees
- high percentage of patients with severe co-morbidities
- high level of expectation from patients regarding the quality of care provided by academic hospitals
- high percentage of innovative therapies with sometimes limited long time results in the context of clinical studies or intention to treat trials

5.3 CRITICAL INCIDENT REPORTING SYSTEM

In the industry, registration or recording of so called critical incidents is a well established procedure to identify systematically errors and errors in the system. The gathered information is submitted a standardized analysis and strategies are derived to prevent or avoid errors or at least their frequency. During the last years, critical incident reporting systems were increasingly established in health care systems. Very often, anesthesiology departments were leading and transferred knowledge and experience won by the industry to the medical setting [4].

In health care systems, **critical incidents** are defined as all situations, actions or circumstances which may decrease patients' safety. Critical incidents are different from accidents or near-accidents (near-misses). Their potential for compromising patients' safety is obviously. Accidents permanently or transitory affect patients' health whereas near-misses per definition do not. Both events are therefore differentiated by the outcome. However, the line between accidents and near-misses is sometimes difficult to draw because the effects may only become obvious after some time delay. As an example, it is well known that intraoperatives periods of hypotension may cause postoperative mnestic alterations such as difficulties to concentrate. However, the individual level of tolerance for periods of hypotension shows a great variety and it is therefore very difficult to predict their impact. This example shows that it is very important that normal limits or, better, limits of normality are defined *a priori*. Every crossing of the limits has then to be regarded as a safety-relevant incident, a so-called critical incident. This requires an anticipating work style and a long process of teaching and learning.

Ten years ago, safety of patients was not a big issue. Only few pioneers in few hospitals were dealing with the subject. The report "To Err is Human: building a safer health care system" published by the American Institute of Medicine in 1999 [9] induced a process of change and had an impressive impact on hospital policies. Today, most American health care providers are dealing with measures to increase patients' safety [10] and Europe is catching up.

5.3.1. Theoretical Basics

The Institute of Medicine National Roundtable on Health Care Quality differentiated three different categories of quality problems during treatment [2]:

- underuse
- overuse
- misuse

Misuse problems are defined as preventable complications of an appropriate treatment and occur with great frequency. If the complication is not identified and treated then the criteria of an erroneous act are met. Misuse is therefore different from error but they are tightly linked. Misuse problems are often obvious to the patient. Consequently, they are least accepted and may cause strong emotional reactions [10].

Overuse problems are also very common and are usually tightly linked with indications for treatments: Patients receive treatments without the right or without any indication. Examples are overuse of antibiotics and inappropriate surgical or endoscopic interventions. Health care service is provided under circumstances in which its potential for harm exceeds the possible benefit. Overuse causes therefore unnecessary risks for patients and health care providers. In contrast to overuse, **underuse** problems are the failure to provide health care service under circumstances in which its potential for benefit exceeds the possible harm. Examples are withheld of treatments for hypertension or acute myocardial infarction and missing immunizations for patients at risk.

Misuse, underuse and overuse problems are sometimes easily identified by people not specialized in health care. Hence, they have a major impact on the public perception of health care providers' quality of treatment. Within health care systems, misuse problems are often the major focus to improve quality of service. Underuse and overuse are much harder to recognize and therefore the true challenge of clinical risk management.

The confrontation with critical situations is part of the daily clinical work of physicians even if they think it does not [1]. The personal experience with accidents and near-misses is limited. Accidents and near-misses are usually not happening out of the nowhere but were often preceded by a much larger number of critical incidents with similar causes. The values of critical incidents are not only that their frequency is much higher – and therefore also the available data – but also that the patients' outcomes are not affected. Hence, talking about them, analyzing them and making the conclusions public pose no legal risk for health care workers and hospitals.

The quantitative relation of critical deviations from normal operation is visually describes by the Iceberg-model (Figure 1) [15]. The steepness of the iceberg, respectively the exact quantitative proportion of critical incidents compared to accidents and near-misses is unknown. Theoretical models in aviation industry assume a factor of ten between each step. This would signify that one accident is preceded by 10 near-misses, 100 critical incidents and 1000 minor errors/flaws with similar causes or circumstances. A critical incident reporting system yields gaining access to this valuable database and to the knowledge and experience made by persons who interrupted the cause-and-effect chain, thus preventing accidents and near-misses from happening. According to the Iceberg-model, all incidents except accidents should be reported. They are sometimes also called safety-relevant incidents because the term incorporates more than only critical incidents.

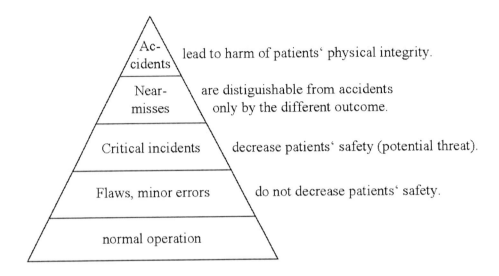

Figure 1. Iceberg model.

The principal concepts of a critical incident reporting system are that the reporting person gets the opportunity to communicate safety-relevant incidents without fearing negative personal consequences and that the information is shared within the department or institution. Essential is also that the reporting person very often prevented an accident by taking appropriate countermeasures. These systems are therefore also denominated "trouble report systems" [7]. The analysis of reported safety-relevant incidents can consequently be used to improve patient safety by two ways: First, causes and causative factors, which led to the incident, are identified. Second, preventive factors and/or solution strategies are given with the trouble report: Which intervention prevented that the patient was harmed? An analysis of accidents is very often less informative because countermeasures or strategies were not effective. The results of such analyses are therefore sometimes only of theoretical value. In safety-relevant incidents, the selected strategies did already prove that they are of practical value. Their potential to reduce risks is therefore much greater. A critical incident reporting system should aim at getting information from all possibly involved people. Every reporter is accepted as expert in his working environment and should be invited to suggest measures to increase patients' safety.

Worldwide, several different reporting systems have been established in health care. These systems

- are obligatory or voluntary.
- are anonymous, confidential or open.
- are supervised internally or externally.
- differ in the way feedback is given to the reporting persons.

All reporting systems have in common that willingness to report decreases when personal consequences are feared. Anonymous reporting systems warrant the highest level of safety for the reporting person and are therefore very often favored [8]. The level of safety is further increased by limiting the number of people with right to access the database. Typically, the heads of the department and the hospital should have no access although their supports for the system are essential. It is therefore obvious that the critical incident task force should work independently from their supervisors.

A critical incident reporting system lives from the number of reports. People tend to report more frequently if they are informed about the reported incidents on a regular base and if consequences derived from the reports are obvious. The long term goal of a critical incident reporting system as a tool of clinical risk management is sustaining the development of a culture of error. Ideally, personal error perception should replace a culture of blame. In this context, it is very important that critical incidents are not communicated as individual failures but as an information pool open to everybody. The analysis of the received information should aim to identify system factors, which facilitate or promote errors. These could be organizational factors, such as availability of interpreters or need for specific training, logistic/technical factors, such as availability or functionality of a certain equipments, and human factors, such as deficits in communication or strong hierarchy. The premise is that complex organizations increase the capacity of an individual to achieve higher goals but that the complexity also introduces sources of error that are not directly attributable to individual (see Table) [16].

Table. Factors influencing the likelihood of incidents in complex health care organizations [modified from 16]

Factors increasing the likelihood of incidents	number of individuals (departments) involved in the care of a patient
	complexity of the tasks involved in the care of a patient
	high status distinction among professional groups, between men and women and social or ethnic groups
	high environmental pressure on an organization to achieve targets that are not directly linked to quality of care
	high organizational pressure to achieve goals that are not directly linked to quality of care
	high discrepancy between the goals of an organization and the funds available
Factors lowering the likelihood of incidents	high emphasis on arrangements for formal communication
	easy identification of an individual as responsible for coordinating the care of a patient
	promotion of the role of individuals to deliver high quality care and increase patient safety
	high formalization and standardization of key tasks (e.g., disinfection, drug administration, resuscitation)
	high organizational and individual commitment to decrease the number and seriousness of adverse events

Hospitals are typical representatives for complex organizations. They incorporate a network of different, specialized departments, which often work in seclusion with sometimes numerous sub-specialized sub-departments. In this working environment, momentous decisions are made, which may have a major impact on following treatment. The operating theatre is a typical example. It is one of the key resources and most important cost driver in hospitals. Here, the work schedule is very dynamic and process oriented. At the same time, working individuals are occasionally and sometimes even systematically deprived of important information. Very often, they have a well-defined duty and their freedom of decision is constricted although their decisions influence patients' integrity and outcome [13]. It is therefore obvious that errors occurring in complex organizations should not be attributed to individual ignorance, incompetence and amorality but that a systematic risk management should focus on identification of organizational factors, which induced, aggravated or negatively influenced the adverse event or its seriousness [3;5;14;16].

5.3.2. Requirements for Implementing a Critical Incident Reporting System

A critical incident reporting system can be implemented on a local or regional (national) basis. It is true that analyses of reports are sometimes of general interest and the results should therefore be available for as many health care workers as possible. Ideally, a local incident reporting system should be combined and connected with a national database. This article focuses on the role of a local risk management, whose institutionalization should stand in first line. The above mentioned complexity of high quality health care organizations produces very often special local conditions. The reported incidents should therefore be analyzed by specialists who are familiar with these special local conditions. This knowledge is very often important to implement successfully countermeasures. This local critical incident reporting system should fulfill several prerequisites:

- The critical incident reporting system has to be supported in an active way by the heads of the departments and the hospital management.
- The task force critical incident should get the status of an autonomous work group to warranty the highest possible independence from superior authorities. This increases the willingness to report.
- The heads of the departments and the hospital management should guarantee all reporting individuals exemption from punishment.
- The critical incident reporting system should aim at highest possible anonymity.
- Reporting should be on a voluntary basis.
- The task force critical incident should consist of representatives of all involved departments and professional categories directly or indirectly involved in the care of the patients. Also, all hierarchies within professional groups should be represented.
- Members of the task force should all be specialists in their fields with the according competence.
- The task force should have the power to implement changes or to delegate specified tasks to ensure changes for improving patients' safety (e.g., algorithms, standard

operating procedures, standing instructions, initialization or improvement of training).

- The critical incident reporting system should be open to everybody in the sense that all professionals involved in the care of patients should have the possibility to report.
- One requirement of a critical incident reporting system is therefore that individuals willing to report have access to the reporting system. A possible technical solution is to use a web-based or intranet-based platform.
- The analyses of the reports should be done without time lag and performed in a structured way.
- The staff should be informed on a regular base about the contents of the reports. The information can be given as informal letters, news announcements or during grand rounds. The consequences initiated due to the reports should be communicated to stimulate further the reporting.
- Consequences should primarily focus on organizational and systematic errors.

As mentioned above, reports entered into a critical incident reporting system very often already include analyses of causes and causative factors, which led to the incidents, and hints for preventive factors and/or solution strategies. It is therefore very important that the reporting health care worker gets the opportunity to express all ideas connected to the critical incident. This can be realized by including an appropriate free-text field into the reporting system.

CONCLUSION

Critical incidents are defined as all situations, actions or circumstances which may decrease patients' safety. They happen every day in a great number and the number further increases when the work environment is as complex as in healthcare organizations. The principal concepts of a critical incident reporting system are that the reporting person gets the opportunity to communicate critical incidents without fearing negative personal consequences and that the information is shared within the department or institution.

The first and most important step during implementation of an anonymous critical incident reporting system into healthcare high risk organizations is the implicit support by the responsible managements. Already indifference from their side, regarding the project may prove to be not only counterproductive but disastrous. The attitude of the management is well registered by the staff and has a major impact on the willingness to report. Another obligatory prerequisite is that the work group clinical risk management works independently and is not constrained by directives. The autonomy of the work group should be made transparent to everybody. The management should not have access to the database of critical incident reports. The superiors are informed by the work group if necessary. Due to this status of the work group, the critical incident reports are comparable to confessional secrets. The work group should analyze the critical incident reports on a regular base using standardized protocols. Consequences taken because of reported events should be made public to increase the willingness to report. They should focus on identification of organizational factors, which induced, aggravated or negatively influenced the adverse event or its seriousness.

Using this approach, the implementation of a critical incident reporting system is a valuable tool for healthcare high risk organizations to improve patients' safety, staffs' satisfaction with their work and to reduce financial and intangible risks for the institution.

REFERENCES

[1]   Adams H. "Where there is error, may we bring truth." A misquote by Margaret Thatcher as she entered No 10, Downing Street in 1979. Anaesthesia 2005; 60: 274-7.

[2]   Chassin MR, Galvin RW, National Roundtable on Health Care. The urgent need to improve health care quality. Institute of Medicine National Roundtable on Health Care. JAMA 1998; 280: 1000-5.

[3]   Classen DC, Kilbridge PM. The roles and responsibility of physicians to improve patient safety within health care delivery systems. Acad Med 2002; 77: 963-72.

[4]   Gaba DM. Anaesthesiology as a model for patient safety in health care. BMJ 2000; 320: 785-8.

[5]   Grout JR. Preventing medical errors by designing benign failures. Jt Comm J Qual Saf 2003; 29: 354-62.

[6]   Hansis ML, Hart D, Becker-Scharzt k, Hansis DE. Medizinische Behandlungsfehler. Gesundheitsberichterstattung des Bundes 2001; 4: 8.

[7]   Hofinger G, Walaczek H. Das Bewusstsein schärfen. Dtsch Arztebl 2003; 100: A2848-9

[8]   Hübler M, Möllemann A, Eberlein-Gonska M, Regner M, Koch T. Anonymous critical incident reporting system in anaesthesiology. Results after 18 months. Anaesthesist 2006; 55: 133-41.

[9]   Kohn LT. To err is human: building a safer health care system. 2000; National Academy Press, Washington, DC.

[10]   Leape LL, Berwick DM. Five years after To Err Is Human: what have we learned. JAMA 2005; 293: 2384-90.

[11]   Möllemann A, Eberlein-Gonska M, Koch T, Hübler M. Clinical risk management. Implementation of an anonymous error registration system in the anesthesia department of a university hospital. Anaesthesist 2005; 54: 377-84.

[12]   Singleton RJ, Ludbrook GL, Webb RK, Fox MA. The Australian Incident Monitoring Study. Physical injuries and environmental safety in anaesthesia: an analysis of 2000 incident reports. Anaesth Intensive Care 1993; 21: 659-63.

[13]   St. Pierre M, Hofinger G, Buerschaper C, Grapengeter M, Harms H, Breuer G, Schuttler J. Simulator-based modular human factor training in anesthesiology. Concept and results of the module "Communication and Team Cooperation". Anaesthesist 2004; 53: 144-52.

[14]   Staender S, Davies J, Helmreich B, Sexton B, Kaufmann M. The anaesthesia critical incident reporting system: an experience based database. Int J Med Inform 1997; 47: 87-90.

[15]   Staender S. Incident reporting as a tool for error analysis in medicine. Z Arztl Fortbild Qualitatssich 2001; 95: 479-84.

[16] West E. Organisational sources of safety and danger: sociological contributions to the study of adverse events. Qual Health Care 2000; 9: 120-6.

In: Dresden Teamwork Concept for Medical…
Editor: Axel R. Heller

ISBN 978-1-60692-307-8
© 2009 Nova Science Publishers, Inc.

Chapter 7

LESSONS LEARNED FROM RISK MANAGEMENT IN ANESTHESIA

Angela Möllemann, Susanne C. Heller and Matthias Hübler
Department of Anesthesiology & Critical Care Medicine,
University Hospital Carl Gustav Carus, University of Technology, Dresden, Germany

ABSTRACT

A local critical incidents reporting system (CIRS) was implemented in the Department of Anesthesiology and Intensive Care of the University Hospital Dresden in 2003. During a observation period of 18 months 162 anonymous reports were received. As expected from the distribution of the number of cases most dispatches came from elective day shift surgery ($73.4\pm4.4\%$) covering $80.3\pm1.0\%$ of procedures (p=0.054). Distribution of error messages showed a relative overweight of vital emergency surgery. While $7.8\pm0.5\%$ of total cases were emergency procedures $13.8\pm2.3\%$ of CIRS messages were related to that type of surgery (p=0.01), insinuating a higher hazard likelihood. This calculation, however might be flawed by the fact that the willingness to report emergency problems is higher.

The most common errors concerned airway and ventilation management, followed by errors in fluid and cardio-vascular management. The main causes were distraction, lack of experience, specific training and communication deficits. The confidence in the anonymity of the reporting system was very high. Following the analysis of the reports, several revisions of the workflow were implemented, e.g., definition of standards or specific training programs. The article discusses the different type of errors occurring and possible countermeasures. Further key elements to be considered during start- up and the initial phase of a local Critical Incident Reporting System and lessons learned are further reviewed.

INTRODUCTION

While critical incident reporting systems have been widely implemented in industry, the healthcare system still remains at the very beginning. Anesthesia departments in many institutions lead the way towards patient safety [1-5]. Aims of such reporting systems are systematic uncovering of safety relevant and critical incidents followed by analysis and subsequent derivation of solutions or strategies of avoidance.

Within the healthcare system worldwide distinct reporting systems have been implemented [6]. The latter are either obligatory or voluntary, anonymous, confidential or open, and are run by internal or external working groups and differ regarding their internal and external feedback. In the Dept. of Anesthesiology and Intensive Care Medicine a critical incident reporting system was implemented as described in chapter 6 [5]. Within the internal working group, which meets on a regular basis it was decided to chose a anonymous, non-punitive system.

The present chapter describes the incidents, analyses, and solutions of a 18 month period from April 2003 until September 2004 in an university teaching anesthesia department during which more than 30.000 anesthesias were performed with 82 physicians (10 consultants, 30 staff anesthetists and 42 residents) and 99 nurses, regularly in 32 up to 45 operating theaters or intervention rooms.

CRITICAL INCIDENT DATA ACQUISITION

Results were obtained by analysis of the anonymous dispatches from the CIRS. Error messages were generated by all members of the clinic (doctors and nurses), by means of a self developed scanner readable questionnaire, which now is migrated to an intranet based system. The development of the feedback form implemented the **Man- Technology- Organization** (MTO) concept [5;7] and additionally allows information on the initial situation/ scenario (time, urgency, initial health status) as well as potential human, technical, or organizational sources of error (Figure 1). Further it was asked for an assessment of severity and preventability. The optional input of a free text provides a detailed presentation. Since it is known, that too complex questionnaires or too low user friendliness is the cause for failure of already implemented CIRS [8], our report form was kept rather short.

As already stated, the collection period amounted to a total of 18 months. With start of the reporting system it was established that, every 6 months, the reports would be systematically analyzed and categorized and would be made available to the employees during a regular lecture. Feed back of results is one key point keeping the interest by the employees and assure to a higher degree continuous submission of reports [8]. The period of 6 months was chosen to guarantee a adequate number of messages suitable for categorization and further statistical evaluation, and, likewise increased anonymity. With respect to the iceberg model (detailed representation in chapter 6) the obtained distribution represents a surrogate for expectable misses and near- misses [9].

The events were analyzed in terms of their relative frequency (reference point was the current 6-month period).

NEAR- MISSES AND CRITICAL INCIDENTS REPORTED

A total of 162 anonymous reports were encountered. They were spread evenly throughout the collection period. The reporting behaviour was continuous and stable over time. It appeared, however, that the willingness for submission of messages directly increased after information sessions.

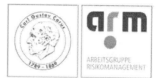

University Hospital Carl Gustav Carus Dresden
Dept of Anesthesiology and Intensive Care Medicine
Head: Prof. Dr. Thea Koch

Critical Incident Reporting System

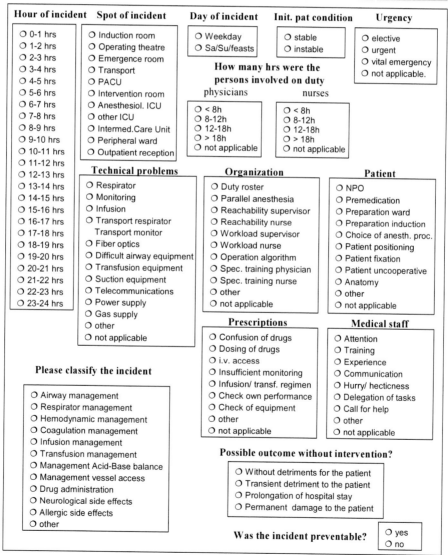

Hour of incident	Spot of incident	Day of incident	Init. pat condition	Urgency
O 0-1 hrs	O Induction room	O Weekday	O stable	O elective
O 1-2 hrs	O Operating theatre	O Sa/Su/feasts	O instable	O urgent
O 2-3 hrs	O Emergence room			O vital emergency
O 3-4 hrs	O Transport	**How many hrs were the**		O not applicable.
O 4-5 hrs	O PACU	**persons involved on duty**		
O 5-6 hrs	O Intervention room	physicians	nurses	
O 6-7 hrs	O Anesthesiol. ICU	O < 8h	O < 8h	
O 7-8 hrs	O other ICU	O 8-12h	O 8-12h	
O 8-9 hrs	O Intermed.Care Unit	O 12-18h	O 12-18h	
O 9-10 hrs	O Peripheral ward	O > 18h	O > 18h	
O 10-11 hrs	O Outpatient reception	O not applicable	O not applicable	
O 11-12 hrs				

O 12-13 hrs	**Technical problems**	**Organization**	**Patient**
O 13-14 hrs	O Respirator	O Duty roster	O NPO
O 14-15 hrs	O Monitoring	O Parallel anesthesia	O Premedication
O 15-16 hrs	O Infusion	O Reachability supervisor	O Preparation ward
O 16-17 hrs	O Transport respirator	O Reachability nurse	O Preparation induction
O 17-18 hrs	Transport monitor	O Workload supervisor	O Choice of anesth. proc.
O 18-19 hrs	O Fiber optics	O Workload nurse	O Patient positioning
O 19-20 hrs	O Difficult airway equipment	O Operation algorithm	O Patient fixation
O 20-21 hrs	O Transfusion equipment	O Spec. training physician	O Patient uncooperative
O 21-22 hrs	O Suction equipment	O Spec. training nurse	O Anatomy
O 22-23 hrs	O Telecommunications	O other	O other
O 23-24 hrs	O Power supply	O not applicable	O not applicable
	O Gas supply		
	O other	**Prescriptions**	**Medical staff**
	O not applicable	O Confusion of drugs	O Attention
		O Dosing of drugs	O Training
Please classify the incident		O i.v. access	O Experience
		O Insufficient monitoring	O Communication
O Airway management		O Infusion/ transf. regimen	O Hurry/ hecticness
O Respirator management		O Check own performance	O Delegation of tasks
O Hemodynamic management		O Check of equipment	O Call for help
O Coagulation management		O other	O other
O Infusion management		O not applicable	O not applicable
O Transfusion management			
O Management Acid-Base balance		**Possible outcome without intervention?**	
O Management vessel access			
O Drug administration		O Without detriments for the patient	
O Neurological side effects		O Transient detriment to the patient	
O Allergic side effects		O Prolongation of hospital stay	
O other		O Permanent damage to the patient	

Was the incident preventable?	O yes
	O no

Figure 1. Print out representation of the intranet based Critical incident reporting sheet © by task force Risk Management (ARM) University Hospital of Dresden, Germany

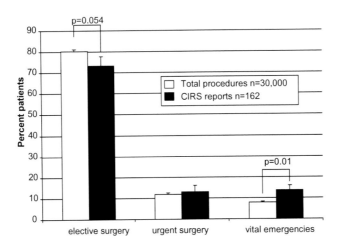

Figure 2. Relative comparison between the distribution of CIRS messages and total cases performed over surgical urgency classes; absolute caseload is given in numbers.

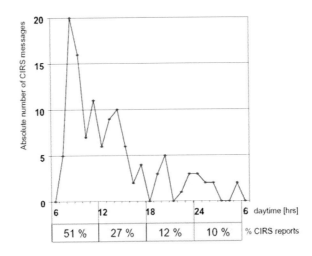

Figure 3. Daytime distribution of CIRS reports independent of urgency.

The largest number of critical incident reports was related to elective daytime surgery (figures 2 & 3). However, the relative proportion was lower than expected when compared to total case load: In urgent surgery no differences were found, while in emergency cases significantly more incidents were reported. This picture is confirmed by the daytime spreading of messages. The early peak may be attributed to normal workload distribution over time with the start of at least 32 operating theatres at 7:30 a.m.

The number of reported technical problems was relatively low (table 1). Additionally, these technical problems were often wrongly classified by the reporting person and actual operating or application errors were masked (e.g., the cancellation of the respirator self test was followed by a non-functional state of the device).

Table 1. Relative number of reports on technical and organizational errors during three 6 month observation periods

Technical errors	Observation periods		
	I (42)	II (67)	III (53)
Respirator	16% (7)	10% (7)	9% (5)
Monitoring	21% (9)	3%[a] (2)	0%[a] (0)
Infusion device	16% (7)	10% (7)	6% (3)
Intubation equipment	2% (1)	3% (2)	4% (2)
Telecommunications	0% (0)	4% (3)	2% (1)
Suction device	5% (2)	0% (0)	0% (0)
Difficult airway equipment	2% (1)	1% (1)	2% (1)
Transfusion facilities	0% (0)	1% (1)	6% (3)
Power supply	5% (2)	0% (0)	0% (0)
Central gas supply	5% (2)	0% (0)	0% (0)
Organization /Duty roster			
Affected physical fitness	2% (1)	3% (2)	4% (2)
Continued shift >12 h	5% (2)	4% (3)	6% (3)
Continued shift >18 h	2% (1)	1% (1)	4% (2)
Continued shift >24 h	0% (0)	0% (0)	0% (0)
Fatigue due to duty roster	2% (1)	1% (1)	0% (0)
Defaulting breaks	2% (1)	1% (1)	2% (1)
More than 2 ORs per nurse	2% (1)	0% (0)	0% (0)

Absolute values in brackets. [a]Significant vs. observation period I.
Observation periods I Apr-Sept 2003; II Oct 2003-Mar2004; III Apr-Sep 2004.

The organization of service very rarely was deemed crucial (table 1) and only in a few cases subjectively reduced physical fitness was considered relevant. Misjudgment of the situation, however, was the most frequently mentioned error within training issues (table 2), insinuating that due to lack of experience the severity of incidents were underestimated and / or the team was not capable to safely perform the appropriate therapeutic measures.

The high number of reports related to incorrect dosage of medications was almost exclusively with regard to propofol and vecuronium. In the case of propofol mostly arithmetic errors occurred (confusion between 1% and 2% propofol, calculation with a wrong body weight or puzzling milliliters and milligrams). Vecuronium was almost exclusively misdosed in pediatrics (confusion with rocuronium).

The individual is very likely to play the key role in all critical events whether it is that personal awareness and the following solving strategies avert disasters, or that individual acts or omissions favor critical events. A clear separation from organizational failures is often neither possible nor desirable, since otherwise the development and formulation of preventive strategies are rendered difficult. Table 3 shows the reported human factors. Almost half of all reports concerned insufficient team awareness.

Table 2. Relative number of reports on errors regarding organization of service and training deficits over three 6 month observation periods

Organization of service	Observation periods		
	I (42)	II (67)	III (53)
Loss of information	21% (9)	7%* (5)	13% (7)
Lack of experience	26% (11)	19% (13)	25% 13)
Default NPO	2% (1)	6% (4)	0% (0)
Insufficient preparation on ward	2% (1)	0% (0)	0% (0)
Insufficient preparation of anesthesia induction procedure	2% (1)	1% (1)	2% (1)
Error by hurry/ hecticness	12% (5)	4% (3)	6% (3)
Lacking utilization of existing human resources	2% (1)	1% (1)	4% (2)
Erroneous task delegation	0% (0)	0% (0)	8% (4)
Lacking leadership by consultant	16% (7)	6% (4)	6% (3)
Default availability of consultant	0% (0)	3% (2)	4% (2)
Default communication	12% (5)	9% (6)	13% (7)
Training deficits			
Misjudgment of situation	33% (14)	22% (15)	26% (14)
Lack of specific training physician	19%[a] (8)	15%[a] (10)	9% (5)
Lack of specific training nurses	2% (1)	3% (2)	4% (2)
Lacking operation algorithm	7% (3)	9% (6)	9% (5)
Unknown operation algorithm	5% (2)	9% (6)	9% (5)
Airway obstruction	12% (5)	19% (13)	4%[b] (2)
Wrong choice of anesthesia procedure	2% (1)	7% (5)	0%[b] (0)
Wrong dosing of drugs	26% (11)	9%* (6)	8%* (4)
Flawed infusions-/transfusion regime	9% (4)	6% (4)	8% (4)
Flawed monitoring	9% (4)	1%* (1)	4% (2)
Erroneous set/ missing alarms	0% (0)	3% (2)	2% (1)
Lacking check of anesthesia equipment	7% (3)	1% (1)	8% (4)
Lacking check of own performance	5% (2)	0% (0)	4% (2)
Flawed previous patient examinations	5% (2)	0% (0)	4% (2)
Difficult anatomy	7% (3)	6% (4)	4% (2)
Flawed utilization of existing auxiliaries	0% (0)	1% (1)	2% (1)

Absolute values in brackets. *Significant vs. observation period I. [s]ignificant vs. lacking specific training nurses; [s]ignificant vs. observation period II. Observation periods I Apr-Sept 2003; II Oct2003-Mar2004; III Apr—Sep2004.

Table 3. Relative number of reports on human errors and preventability over three 6 month observation periods

Human errors	Observation period		
	I (42)	II (67)	III (53)
Attention deficits	35% (15)	45% (30)	44%
Defaulting contraindications	2% (1)	0% (0)	0% (0)
Defaulting prior examinations	5% (2)	0% (0)	4% (2)
Defaulting coexisting disease	2% (1)	3% (2)	9% (5)
Too low level of anesthesia	2% (1)	7% (5)	8% (4)
Missed call for help	7% (3)	1% (1)	4% (2)
Drug confusion	2% (1)	3% (2)	4% (2)
Preventable	95% (40)	96% (64)	100% (53)

Absolute values in brackets. Observation periods: I Apr-Sept 2003; II Oct2003-Mar2004; III Apr—Sep2004.

ACTIONS TAKEN FOR PREVENTION/REDUCTION OF CRITICAL EVENTS

After analysis of the anonymous reports, and taking into account generally known (non-anonymous) incidents (including accidents or near misses) the task force risk management initiated at least 11 larger measures for the prevention or reduction of critical events of which the following three are presented as examples.

- A poster difficult airway, adapted to the local peculiarities, was created including an operation algorithm with devices to secure the airway. This algorithm was posted in all anesthesia workstations. Further, according to the algorithm numerous devices were procured and a mandatory training on regular basis for all medical and nursing staff at phantoms was implemented on regular basis.
- In order to avoid confusion between regional anesthesia catheters and intravenous catheters regarding injected drugs, a compulsory marking of the catheter systems with eye-catching stickers was introduced. The confusion was solely reported on normal wards and intensive care units not managed by the Department of Anesthesia. Figure 4 gives an example of the flyers as issued by the task force.
- Due to several reports on the entry of ferromagnetic objects in the magnetic resonance imaging (MRI) examination room, which had led to threats of patients (fortunately no direct hits) a "MRI procedure and checklist" was created, to be adhered to by patients and employees before entering the room.

In addition, various regulations were issued or technical changes were prompted: During artificial ventilation set lower alarm limit for inspiratory oxygen concentration to 30%; Functional test and drill alert of the resuscitation team at 8:15 a.m. (radio reception of pagers was variable, pagers were taken home after nightshift); Locations of defibrillators on the campus were uniformly marked; Definition of standard minimum content for emergency cases on peripheral wards. Furthermore, to improve communication skills, leadership, teamwork, resource management and decision-making capabilities, a mandatory Crisis-Resource Management (CRM) training in our simulation center (ISIMED) [10] was implemented.

Department of Anesthesiology and Intensive Care Medicine
Head: Prof. Dr. med T. Koch
Task Force Risk Management ©

Phone (0351) 458-2785
Fax: (0351) 458 4336
Email: ane.risikomanagement@uniklinikum-dresden.de

Flyer 3

Identification of regional anesthesia catheters and corresponding feeding lines

The unintentional administration of intravenous drugs into a regional anesthesia catheter is a potentially serious complication. Toxic and ischemic damage to the nervous system may result. Appropriate therapeutic emergency measures after such complications are not known. Similarly, the inadvertent intravenous administration of local anesthetics, planned for injection into regional anesthesia catheters, contributes to morbidity and mortality of patients, as central and cardio- circulatory adverse effects can be expected culminating in respiratory and cardiovascular arrest.

Causes for these unintended injections are the confusing of ampoules in the course of preparing the infusion syringes or puzzling the catheters during the application. The aim must, therefore be to minimize the risk for this confusion. One way to reduce the risk is the color-coded labeling of both, the regional anesthesia catheters and the feeding lines from injection pumps or other patient controlled systems.

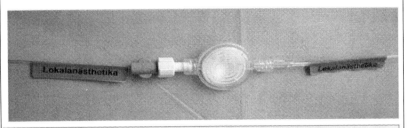

Our critical incident reporting system revealed three messages within the past year, which reported inadvertent connections of syringes and feeding lines filled with local anesthetics with an intravenous line. The Task Force Risk Management is therefore forced to dispose the use of green adhesive labels with the words "Local anesthetics" as a standard. The labels will address both, the peripheral and neuraxial regional anesthesia catheters and must be attached to the immediate vicinity of the coupling hub as well as to all corresponding feeding lines at the end next to the filter (see illustration). The necessary stickers are available in the regional anesthesia chests of drawers. The Task Force is convinced that this measure meets with your approval, and thanks in advance for your support, to keep the implementation phase short and easy.

Literature:
1. Hew CM, Cyna AM, Simmons SW: Avoiding inadvertent injection of drugs of intended for non-epidural use. Anaesth Intensive Care 2003; 31(1): 44-49.
2. Kasaba T, Uehara K, Katsuki H, Ono Y, Takasaki M: Analysis of inadvertent epidural injection of drugs. Masui 2000; 49(12): 1391-94.
3. Peduto VA, Mezzetti D, Gori F: A clinical diagnosis of inadvertent epidural administration of potassium chloride. Eur J Anaesthes 1999; 16(6): 410-12.

Sincerely, Task Force Risk Management   January 2004

Figure 4. Flyer 3 by Task Force Risk Management University Hospital Dresden, Germany, regarding the problem of confusion of regional anesthesia catheters and intravenous access lines.

CRITICAL APPRAISAL OF THE LOCAL CIRS

An anonymous, generally accessible reporting system bears the risk of multiple replays to the same incident by different persons. Such doubles may merely be identified by comparing the respective free text inputs and were, however only very rarely observed. The possibility of multiple nominations should not be considered as a weakness, but a great strength of the system, because a certain situation may be analyzed and assessed by different people from different angles. This facilitates the deduction of general prevention and mitigation strategies, as often already indicated within the free texts.

Relatively speaking, the largest number of reports regarded emergency procedures (Figure 2). This does not mean that actually more incidents happened in these cases, but can also indicate an increased reporting willingness having just encountered the respective critical situation. Likewise, the lack of attention stated in almost half of the cases under no circumstances permits the conclusion that a lack of attention occurs in the daily clinical work with the same frequency. Similarly critical the present cumulative analysis has to be judged. We do not know with absolute certainty, if the observed changes over time represent a true change within daily work or merely reflect a reporting behavior by chance. Consequently, critical efficiency review of the implemented changes it is of eminent importance.

The distinct implementation of technology into daily work increases patient safety, but, likewise, raises various further sources of error. In addition to technical problems these are in first line handling errors, but also the insufficient use of technical possibilities. In this context, ignoring or shutting down alarms is a typical example, not to use technical opportunities to increase patient safety [1].

At first glance, the frequency of mentions of lack of attention and misjudgment of the situation is surprising. Readers being not familiar with the principle of risk management may here assume pure human error. The so-called human errors can at least be divided into 2 types of errors [11]: Slips and mistakes. Slips are unintended and unconscious deviations from expected acts. They are particularly observed when people are emotionally distracted, tired or stressed. They are also the result of a lack of concentration. The recognition of slips itself induces further distraction. Thus, slips often are observed to cumulate within a situation [12]. However, mistakes are genuine errors. They are based on a lack of knowledge, on the lack of the capacity to interpret data or conditions, or on the application of false rules. Stress, fatigue and distraction favor slips, while mistakes, rather, are the result of inadequate training or experience. On closer scrutiny both types of errors shown here are consequences of process or organizational weaknesses and therefore can not be attributed to the individual.

Reports on emergency surgery significantly were overrepresented. The latter scenarios typically favor slips, in particular, when the processes are not optimized. Another indication of shortcomings in the workflow is the frequency of mentions on lack of attention. This is alarming, but also a typical problem immanent to anesthesia, because in clinical practice relatively long periods of stability favoring drop of vigilance may quickly turn into turbulent states. In this regard anesthesia in the same way as aviation has been characterized as: "hours of boredom, minutes of thrill, and seconds of terror" [9]. Despite or even due to the problem of vigilance the, thus, impaired capacity subjectively is not regularly recognized. This is certainly also related to the fact that the admission of fatigue or exhaustion is hardly to be brought into accordance with our professional image [13], even though, many work in the past, could show the opposite [14].

In addition to implementing technical, infrastructural and organizational improvements it should be one objective of the CIRS, to identify errors in knowledge and in rules and to execute appropriate counter measures. They may, for example, consist in formulation of standard operation procedures, of which until now 15 have been set into action. Further, special theoretical training or the implementation of practical exercises, ideally using phantoms or simulators or regular case conferences are a very effective medium and a clear way to overcome typical knowledge errors and to improve skills. In this regard case conferences, however, are a very sensitive area, because the anonymity at least in part may be left. The case selection should, hence, be made very carefully and always presented by a neutral person.

Our daily work is almost exclusively done in the team. Consequently, training and practice of so-called non- technical skills is crucial (see also chapters 4&5), such as communication skills, leadership, teamwork, resource management and decision-making competence [15]. Within a functioning team, process control - regardless of the hierarchical position – should be daily practice. This includes the willingness to give constructive criticism and, personally even harder, to adopt criticism. To promote non- technical skills, particularly Crew Resource Management (CRM) workshops together with psychologists are of eminent value [16]. Therefore, we consciously seek close cooperation with the clinic established simulation center ISIMED [10] (see also chapter 5) which is run by instructors approved by the European Resuscitation Council (ERC).

The most important prerequisite for deducing prevention or mitigation strategies from critical incidents is to develop both, an individual and an institutionalized culture of dealing with error. The aim of our local CIRS is not primarily to analyze extremely rare events, rather, to learn from often experienced security relevant incidents before they reach the disaster level within the iceberg model [9]. These are usually strongly influenced by local conditions so that an effective risk management always should be regionally adapted. By further disseminating the results through a joint action by a multitude of hospitals (e.g., CIRSmedical [17] or PaSOS [18]), smaller structural units and other hospitals may also benefit.

The deduced consequences should reduce the hazard likelihood. For that sake, critical events may neither be experienced nor understood as *individual failures of persons*, because they provide an invaluable pool of information for the identification of *systemic factors and errors*. This knowledge and experience pool is to be utilized and to be provided to the entire department/ scientific community to increase the safety of our patients.

CONCLUSION

An anonymous Critical Incidents Reporting System allows systematic analysis of safety relevant incidents. This requires the development of individual and institutional culture of dealing with error. Derived measures should be focused on training, technical modifications, definition or improvement/ adaptation of standards as well as in communication and teamwork training.

ACKNOWLEDGEMENTS

The Task Force Risk Management/ CIRS besides the authors of this chapter consists of the following individuals without their continuous effort and input this project would not have been possible: Maria Eberlein- Gonska M.D. (Head of Dept. of Quality Management University Hospital, Dresden), Dipl. Ing. Maic Regner (Chief Engineer, Dept. of Anesthesiology and Intensive Care Medicine, UKD), Elisabeth Eickhoff M.D. (Resident in anesthesiology), Siegfried Horter M.D. (Consultant anesthesiologist), Birgit Handrick, Annetta Petrasch (Registered Nurses Anesthesiology).

The Authors are further indebted to the willingness of all staff of the department to report frankly on their own errors and to the Head of the Dept. of Anesthesiology and Intensive Care Medicine/ UKD Prof. Thea Koch M.D. for her unreserved continuous support.

REFERENCES

[1]   Beatty PC, Beatty SF. Anaesthetists' intentions to violate safety guidelines. Anaesthesia 2004 Jun;59(6):528-40.

[2]   Cooper JB, Newbower RS, Kitz RJ. An analysis of major errors and equipment failures in anesthesia management: considerations for prevention and detection. Anesthesiology 1984 Jan;60(1):34-42.

[3]   Gaba DM. Anaesthesiology as a model for patient safety in health care. BMJ 2000 Mar 18;320(7237):785-8.

[4]   Hübler M, Möllemann A, Eberlein-Gonska M, Regner M, Koch T. [Anonymous critical incident reporting system in anaesthesiology. Results after 18 months]. Anaesthesist 2006 Feb;55(2):133-41.

[5]   Möllemann A, Eberlein-Gonska M, Koch T, Hübler M. [Clinical risk management. Implementation of an anonymous error registration system in the anesthesia department of a university hospital]. Anaesthesist 2005 Apr;54(4):377-84.

[6]   To err is human: building a safer health system. Washington D.C.: National Academy Press; 2000.

[7]   Grube C, Schaper N, Graf BM. [Man at risk. Preventive strategies and risk management for patient safety]. Anaesthesist 2002 Apr;51(4):239-47.

[8]   Nyssen AS, Aunac S, Faymonville ME, Lutte I. Reporting systems in healthcare from a case-by-case experience to a general framework: an example in anaesthesia. Eur J Anaesthesiol 2004 Oct;21(10):757-65.

[9]   Rall M, Manser T, Guggenberger H, Gaba DM, Unertl K. [Patient safety and errors in medicine: development, prevention and analyses of incidents]. Anasthesiol Intensivmed Notfallmed Schmerzther 2001 Jun;36(6):321-30.

[10]   Interdisciplinary Medical Simulation Center Dresden, Germany. ISIMED 2008 [cited 2008 Jun 5];Available from: URL: http://www.isimed.info/isimed_/index_eng.html

[11]   Shohania KG, Wald H, Gross R. Understanding medical error and improving patient safety in the in patient setting. Med Clin North Am 2005;86:847-67.

[12] Mackenzie CF, Hu PF, Mahaffrey MA, the LOTAS Group. Group decision-making during trauma patient resuscitation and anesthesia. Human Factors and Ergonomics Society. 1993. p. 372-6.

[13] Williamson JA, Webb RK, Sellen A, Runciman WB, Van der Walt JH. The Australian Incident Monitoring Study. Human failure: an analysis of 2000 incident reports. Anaesth Intensive Care 1993 Oct;21(5):678-83.

[14] Flin R, Fletcher G, McGeorge P, Sutherland A, Patey R. Anaesthetists' attitudes to teamwork and safety. Anaesthesia 2003 Mar;58(3):233-42.

[15] Fletcher GC, McGeorge P, Flin RH, Glavin RJ, Maran NJ. The role of non-technical skills in anaesthesia: a review of current literature. Br J Anaesth 2002 Mar;88(3):418-29.

[16] Müller MP, Hänsel M, Stehr SN, Fichtner A, Weber S, Hardt F, et al. Six steps from head to hand: a simulator based transfer oriented psychological training to improve patient safety. Resuscitation 2007 Apr;73(1):137-43.

[17] German Chamber of Physicians. Reporting and Learning System of German Physicians for Critical Incidents in Medicine. Bundesärztekammer 2008 [cited 2008 Jun 5];Available from: URL: http://www.cirsmedical.de/

[18] German Society of Anesthesiology and Intensive Care Medicine. Patient Safety Optimizing System. DGAI 2008 [cited 2008 Jun 5];Available from: URL: https://www.pasos-ains.de/main.php

In: Dresden Teamwork Concept for Medical…
Editor: Axel R. Heller

ISBN 978-1-60692-307-8
© 2009 Nova Science Publishers, Inc.

Chapter 8

SIX SIGMA – AN INDUSTRIAL MANAGEMENT TOOL TO OPTIMIZE HIGH RISK MEDICAL PROCESSES

Stephan B. Sobottka[1], Jörn Großekatthöfer[2], Swen Günther[2], Axel R. Heller[3] and Detlev Michael Albrecht[4]

[1]Dept. Neurosurgery, [3]Dept. Anesthesiology and Critical Care Medicine, [4]CEO, University Hospital Carl Gustav Carus, [2]Corporate Management and Marketing University of Technology, Dresden, Germany

ABSTRACT

To reach practicable zero- defect quality in hospitals modern management concepts have to be utilized, which must be adapted to clinical peculiarities. Six Sigma is such an innovative management- approach, which seeks perfection by strict avoidance of defects within the workflow. The core of the Six Sigma approach in the hospital is the substantial improvement of medical service processes.

The Six Sigma principle utilizes strategies, which are based on quantitative measurements and which seek to optimize processes, limit deviations or dispersion from the target process. Hence, Six Sigma aims to eliminate errors or quality problems of all kinds. Therefore, well-established techniques in quality management are combined with simple and advanced methods of data analysis and systematic training of staff. With the focus on quality improvement by failure prevention, Six Sigma enables identification of weaknesses in hospital processes and achieving a workable zero- defect quality by using a standardized process- and patient- oriented approach.

For the first time in German health system a pilot project to optimize the preparation for neurosurgery could now show that using the Six Sigma method enhanced patient safety in medical care, while at the same time disturbances in the hospital processes and failure costs could be avoided. Hence, the financial performance of the clinic was improved.

INTRODUCTION

"Primum nil nocere" - "First, no harm" is a central dogma in medical conduct. This includes the continuous efforts of doctors, to frame medical treatment as safe as possible and to avoid unnecessary risks and iatrogenic damage. Risks are preceding hazard potentials of a desired quality. In the case avoidable risks are identified in advance, or even are reduced or eliminated, quality is brought to a higher level. If they, however, remain undetected quality will drop, the safety of patients will be threatened and damage to health or even death may result. Compared to other high-risk areas, such as aviation or nuclear power plants, where adverse events are associated with a high risk potential for a large number of people, safety risks in medicine usually merely concern single patients. The impact on the latter individuals, however, is not less serious.

Neurosurgery in the brain or spinal cord are high-risk medical procedures. Errors, miscalculations and complications can be followed by irreversible damage, such as paralysis, language loss, blindness and memory and personality disorders as well. Due to the high degree of functional complexity of the brain and inter-individual variability of anatomical structures and the localization of eloquent functional areas, today's neurosurgical interventions require extensive preparation and meticulous planning. In this regard a variety of anatomical and functional examinations have to take place and have to be made available to the surgeon beforehand surgery. Only by providing all the necessary operation related information, the existing risks of neurosurgery can be identified and be rated by the physician. Consequently, this way of preparation within the complex environment ensures that even short-term decisions by the surgeon in the operating room only bear a limited risk, for the patient and can be made in his sense. To avoid errors and omissions in the preparation beforehand surgery consistently and permanently, the introduction of an effective risk management system is needed, with the objective of a viable zero- defect quality by continuous improvements. As a pilot project in our department could show, by the use of modern management techniques such as Six Sigma methodology, sustainable improvements in patient safety and, therefore, the best possible conditions for an optimal quality of neurosurgical treatment could be created.

THE SIX SIGMA PHILOSOPHY

Six Sigma was developed by Motorola in the 1980-ies as *Total Quality Management* approach [4]. The Six Sigma principle aims towards strategies, basing on quantitative measurements and tries to optimize processes, deviations or restrict dispersion and to eliminate errors or quality problems of all kinds. Therefore, well-established techniques in quality management are combined with simple and advanced methods of data analysis and systematic training of staff in all organizational levels.

With the focus on quality improvement by failure prevention it is possible to identify weaknesses in the business processes and to reach a workable and zero- defect quality using a standardized process and customer-oriented approach. The philosophy here is to provide products and services with high-quality by targeted translation of the "voice of the customer" into the "language of the process" and by this means to gain efficiency, customer satisfaction, and effectiveness.

In many economic areas achieving business excellence for some time became self-selected standard targeting at a zero- defect level. In areas such as aircraft industry and specifically the production of aircraft turbines, construction of power plants, and medical technology, in particular in life support devices, this is for security reasons mandatory and reached at a high level. In recent years, the Six Sigma philosophy was introduced to a greater extent in banks and insurance companies representing service business.

Design and Content of Six Sigma

Six Sigma was originally a project-management approach developed for production companies, economically meeting the main internal and external customer requirements by lean and efficient processes within the organization [1]. The focuses of Six Sigma are, in particular the three implementation drivers **customer – process – quality**. Within a practicable zero defect quality on the 6σ- level a quality level of 99.99966% (based on a standard normal distribution) is desired. This corresponds with 3.4 defect - if extrapolated – in a million of defect opportunities in products or services. In the Six Sigma language, this means 3.4 DPMO (*Defects Per Million Opportunities*). In smaller quantities or case numbers, defects, consequently, even more affect achievable total quality.

Within that context an defect is defined as a significant deviation from a defined standard. In the medical field these are either key patient or customer requirements, the so-called **CTQs** as **Critical to Quality Characteristics**, the required quality level of patient safety in the framework of risk management, the quality level set by the strategy of the hospital for differentiation from the competitors or the prescribed standards by legal rules. In all four instances, the performance and generation of value, spawned by a certain process, is qualitatively not sufficient on occurrence of defects [13]. The dispersion of characteristic values, as measured by their standard deviation σ around their mean value μ, must therefore be kept as low as possible. In other words, all characteristic values of good quality shall range within a distance from the mean value to the specification limits of $6\ \sigma$. In this regard the patient/customer does not feel the average value, but the variance, that is the deviation from the default, which may hit him hard, personally. The higher the sigma level and consequently the required level of quality, the smaller is the tolerance interval and, thus, the number of allowable errors.

Six Sigma ideally focuses on processes that are high priority and, likewise, usually bear a high defect rate, or at least have a substantial risk of error. Therefore, particularly in clinical risk management Six sigma will be of advantage. As already mentioned, the measure of the reached quality level is the **sigma value**. Besides the *net benefit* generated within the project, which also can be considered as net cost savings or increase in revenue, the sigma value is a key identification and comparative measure within the Six Sigma concept. It represents a general quality indicator which can be calculated for all relevant processes in hospital. All workflows and process results can, hence, be directly compared which each other based on the Sigma value, even if the customer requirements and, thus, the acceptable quality tolerances differ. It is just critical that the calculated value ranges within the defined limits of tolerance for zero- defect quality. In this regard a key misunderstanding of the Six Sigma philosophy must be addressed: The aim is not complete and absolute absence of defects, because within processes this is hardly possible or much too costly. Workable and, thus, also practised zero- defect quality rather ensures that all deviations range within the allowed tolerances, defined by the external or internal customers, the required quality level by clinical risk management for patient safety, by the strategy driven level, or the one formulated by legal requirements.

The Sigma value became a **quantitative measure**, which in practice identifies the achieved level of quality towards zero- defect quality, regarding the individual process, entire departments or the hospital as whole.

IMPROVEMENT PROJECTS CONSIDERING THE DMAIC CYCLE

The project focus of Six Sigma is characterized by a standardized approach, namely the DMAIC cycle with its five phases: *Define, Measure, Analyse, Improve* and *Control*. This project cycle is based on the classic Deming cycle PDCA (*Plan, Do, Check, Act*) and sets off with the measurement and analysis of CTQs representing the essential customer requirements [6].

Figure 1 depicts the typical progress of the DMAIC cycle with examples of instruments from specific Six Sigma projects, as used in practice. Basically, at the beginning of each Six Sigma project, the **project charter** is set up. The latter and the projected effects as net benefit are the basis for the decision on the project start.

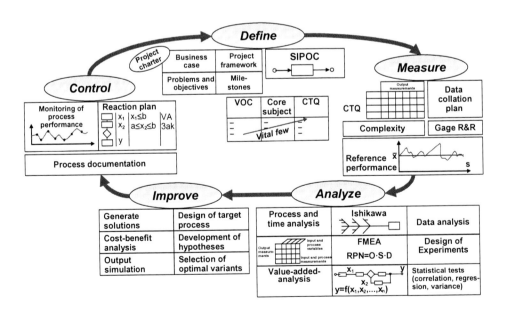

Figure 1. Phases and content of the DMAIC- cycle [13] by courtesy of Prof. A. Töpfer ©

Particularly during the measure and analysis phases advanced mathematical- statistical methods are employed. At the same time, well-known and proven quality management tools, such as failure mode and effect analysis (FMEA), Ishikawa diagram, design of experiments (DOE) and Quality Function Deployment (QFD) are utilized systematically.

During the specific phases of the DMAIC-cycle the following five questions have to be clarified:

1. What is the problem? To answer this question, the main requirements of the customer are to be defined as CTQs. *(Define)*
2. How can the impact be measured? For this purpose relevant impact and result sizes are measured in practice. *(Measure)*
3. What are the causes of the problem? In this phase, the leading causes are analyzed and prioritized based on statistics. *(Analyze)*
4. How can the problem be solved? Based on the analyses improvements or an optimal solution are developed and implemented. *(Improve)*
5. How will the improvement be anchored in practice? It must be ensured that the main causes for the occurrence of the problem are permanently eliminated. *(Control)*

The general approach is to translate a real problem into a statistical problem which then is analyzed for its causes. The obtained statistical problem- solution is checked for its stability in impact, and the optimum solution is then transferred to reality. Further, it is stabilized at a high level by quality assurance measures. In the real project application of the Six Sigma DMAIC cycle, it is not just directly passed once, but it will be jumped back to upstream stages again, depending on the data, identified causes and targeted analyses.

The efficiency and **effectiveness** of a Six Sigma project in the hospital may be rated based on results from **three categories**:

- Success related to increase patient safety, improving medical outcomes and improve satisfaction of patients and other internal and external customers
- Service related in reduction of complexity, in the defect reduction, namely quality improvement, increase productivity and rising employee satisfaction;
- Finance related in shortening the duration of the entire process, in error cost reduction and improvement of the financial results

The results achieved by a Six Sigma project must be calculated against the cost of employee training and project implementation and mark the gained **net benefit**. The calculation of the results achieved is limited to *hard facts,* that means quantifiable results, immediately increasing liquidity and/ or the success of the company, only within a period of twelve months, usually after project completion. On this basis the net benefit of Six Sigma projects on grounds of qualification- and project implementation costs is relatively easy to achieve by a cost-benefit analysis.

ZERO- DEFECT QUALITY AS A REQUIREMENT IN MEDICAL HIGH-RISK AREAS

As international studies suggest, medical treatment errors represent a significant problem in inpatient health care. According to the U.S. Institute of Medicine annually between 44,000 to 98,000 patients in U.S. hospitals die due to medical treatment errors [3]. Adverse events not deriving from the underlying disorder, occur at a frequency of around 2.9% in all hospital patients.

In Germany, data on that topic is not readily available. As reported by the German Council of Experts (SVR) for the Concerted Action in Health care [5], the annual number of suspected and notified treatment errors in Germany range around 40,000. When transferring the frequency and consequences of adverse events from the U.S. studies to German circumstances, in view of the SVR 31,000- 83,000 people would die as a consequence of hospital treatment per year. Considering that about 50% of these cases are preventable in principle, the risk to die in the context of a medical error would be higher than that for dying from colon cancer, breast cancer or traffic accidents [5].

Given the data on the incidence of treatment errors in hospitals and the increasing competition in the health sector, the introduction of zero- defect strategies for medical treatment processes seems useful and necessary. By use of the Six Sigma method it should be possible to increase patient safety in medical care, while by avoiding of failure costs and elimination of disturbances in hospital processes the financial performance of the clinic will improve.

Apart from some projects in the United States and the Netherlands, the Six Sigma methodology has not yet found its way to the health care system [14]. The objective of the project described was to evaluate the suitability of the methodology to optimize safety relevant processes in a medical high-risk area and to compare the extent of reachable quality improvement with the necessary effort.

For that purpose the Six Sigma methodology was applied to the preparation for neurosurgical procedures as a key process with high relevance for patient safety and for optimization of the workflow at the Neurosurgery Clinic of the University of Dresden, Germany. This project is the first known and published Six Sigma application in the German hospital sector.

In neurosurgery next to a prudent and accurate surgical handling the careful and sound surgical planning represents an essential success factor, significantly affecting patient safety. Besides general preparations for surgery in vital organs this includes the reliable and accurate provision of key technical equipment. The surgery microscope is one of those devices, facilitating visualization of important anatomic structures in brain surgery. Further pieces of equipment are the neuro- navigation for precise operational planning of access routes, endoscopes for performing minimally invasive surgery, lasers or ultrasound dissectors to facilitate tumor resection, intra operative imaging techniques, such as 3D- ultrasound, CT or MRI, to control the extent of resection in brain tumor surgery or electrophysiological and functional examinations to identify and monitor functionally important brain areas and structures.

But also missing and incorrect documents in preparation for surgery increase the likelihood that in the OR complex short-term decisions must be taken at respective risk. This is related with a basically avoidable restriction of patient safety.

Hospital Portrait, the Initial Situation and Project Team

In the Clinic of Neurosurgery of the University of Dresden each year about 2,000 surgical procedures in the brain, the spinal cord or peripheral nerves are performed. For that purpose three neurosurgical operating rooms are available.

The hospital disposes of 40 normal ward beds, eight intermediate-care beds, six intensive care beds in an interdisciplinary surgical intensive care unit, furthermore, since 2004 one monitoring unit with four epilepsy surgery beds. The medical staff consists of the Hospital Director Prof. Dr. G. Schackert, six neurosurgical consultants, two staff neurosurgeons and ten residents.

The focus of surgical activity in Dresden is set to the field of brain tumors, including the interdisciplinary treatment of complex skull base tumors and brain tumors in children, open and neuroradiologic- interventional treatment of aneurysms and arteriovenous malformations, functional stereotactic neurosurgery, epilepsy surgery, the surgical treatment of spinal column disorders, chronic pain syndromes and the treatment of diseases of the peripheral nerves. The clinic offers the care of a Tertiary referral Hospital including all neurosurgical emergencies (traumatic brain injury, bleeding, subarachnoid bleeding, acute paraplegia, nerve injuries, hydrocephalus, tumors, paralysis, child and adult emergencies) and is available as a reference centre for immediate and emergency consultation for CT and MRI images to all surrounding hospitals and practitioners around the clock. According to the range of services of the clinic, there are a multitude of special consultation hours.

Following the successful introduction of a pro- active risk management system in the hospital a risk portfolio of all medical service processes was created by means of a comprehensive systematic employee survey [7-9]. The medical staff classified the surgery preparation and planning as a success relevant and in the highest degree safety relevant process, with a strong improvement potential. Because of the outstanding importance of **preparation for surgery** determining the success of neurosurgery, this process was favored by the hospital management and medical clinic employees to be subject of a Six Sigma **pilot project**.

The pilot project was carried out with intensive care and support of the research group at the Chair of Corporate Management and Marketing (LfMU) at the University of Technology Dresden. This group in the past has focused and specialized on the topic of Six Sigma in research and teaching as well as in cooperation projects in business practice.

The Six Sigma project team consisted of representatives of all professional stakeholder groups participating in the process, including the respective process owners and doctors, surgical staff, nurses and technicians. This was mainly due to the high complexity of the process of surgical preparation. In the project with a total of five workshops 5-7 employees of the Clinic of Neurosurgery were involved in each one. The project partner LfMU added counselors with significant experience in both, the field of Six Sigma (black belt/ green belt) as well as in hospital management. This enabled well and quick solving of interface problems, which could e.g., derive from the specifics of the hospital system or the Six Sigma methods used [2;10;11].

PROJECT PROGRESS AND RESULTS

The planning and implementation of Six Sigma pilot project was based on the standardized approach of DMAIC cycle with the five phases: Define, Measure, Analyze, Improve and Control. In addition to achieving optimal patient safety, besides others, the number of preoperative days without treatment, representing a major cost driver, was in the focus of the analysis.

At the start of the Six Sigma project a **project charter** was set up for clear definition of the project objectives. Problem priorities are the timely completion of daily surgical procedure schedule and the surgical patient record. The aim of this project comprises a total of four points. From the clinical viewpoint, the increase in patient safety/ satisfaction and increasing employee satisfaction on the basis of fewer errors/ omissions and avoided treatment errors were sought as major non- monetary value adding components.

From the economic viewpoint, in particular the reduction of preoperative hospital stay, the avoidance of double examinations as well as minimizing the patient waiting time in the operating room was of interest. The net benefit, namely the net savings, were estimated around € 90,000. The determination of the latter is based on a detailed comparison of project costs, cost savings and revenue increases.

To gain the largest possible leverage effect, the boundaries for the project were selected relatively spacious. Thus, the inspection of the process starts in the outpatient reception and ends at the beginning of surgery. The involvement of different stakeholders, such as nursing and surgical-technical staff allowed a comprehensive analysis of the surgical preparation process in the Department of Neurosurgery. The list of project participants also sharing responsibility is accordingly extensive. For the implementation of the project, which started in July 2006, a period of 6 months was estimated.

Next to the definition of the project charter and the "official start" of the Six Sigma project a demarcation of the process to be analyzed ensued on "high level". Therefore, in the **define-phase** a SIPOC analysis (see Figure 2) was performed, in which the input-output relations by the (internal) suppliers to the (internal) customers were roughly outlined.

As quickly appeared, the actual process of surgical preparation on "high level" includes a total of 6 steps. For the smooth implementation of surgery preparation a number of suppliers are required that provide inputs "in due time at the right place". At the same time, the outputs of the individual process steps cover a relatively large number of customers with very different requirements/ needs. While e.g., the anesthetist demands a correct and complete medical history, the surgical technical staff attaches importance to a binding equipment plan with individual patient related surgery data/ schedule.

The SIPOC analysis represents the source for the derivation of the key customer/ patient requirements within the VOC CTQ analysis. By this means originating from the "unfiltered" voice of the customer (VOC) the essential and measurable criteria (CTQs - Critical to Quality Characteristics) related to the workflow processes to be improved were concluded. From the fairly extensive VOC list the 6 key customer requirements (vital few) were filtered and specified as CTQs. According to the initial assessment by the project team the specified target levels were rather challenging. The CTQ "complete OR schedule no later than 2 working days (48 h) prior to OP-start" for example was not reached at the present project state, since the completion of the surgical schedule by default took place not before the preoperative day. Accomplishment of the CTQ "100% completeness of the surgical record by 4 p.m. on the eve of surgery" was on the opposite deemed most likely. In this context various improvement activities were already done prior to the Six Sigma project.

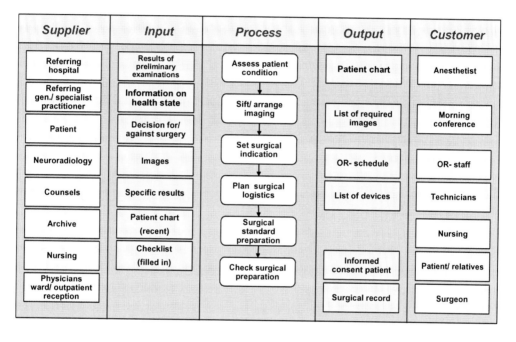

Figure 2. SIPOC analysis.

At the beginning of the **measure-phase** based on the identified CTQs the main output, process, and input measures were deduced. After the project CTQ-output indicator analysis the six identified CTQs could be mapped by of a total of nine output measures Y_i. In this regard the CTQ "100% documentation of changes in the OR schedule" correlated moderately with the output- indicator Y_{41} "Degree of completion of the OR- schedule on eve of surgery" and strong with Y_{42} "Rate of communicated changes in the OR schedule". The assessment of the strength of relationship based on subjective perceptions/ experience in the team, were incorporated in the further project work as basic assumptions.

For the measurement of the 9 Ys a total of 4 checklists were used. In the two measured phases (measure and control phase), they were filled in each over a period of 20 days by doctors and nurses. The first measuring phase to determine the reference performance took place in July/ August 2006.

For each output indicator a sigma value was calculated based on the DPMO formula. Preceding each measurement phase a detailed data collecting plan was established in which the 9 key performance indicators were specified in terms of the 6 questions: What?, Why?, Who?, How?, When? and Where? These operational and therefore precise definitions of single indicators were of particular importance for the quality of the measurements. As in industrial business the use of unambiguous terms is a prerequisite for a common process understanding.

Figure 3, gives the DPMO and **sigma results of the first measuring phase** at a glance. The average quality of German industry with approximately 10,000 DPMO or 3.8σ and the level of best-in-class companies, with about 30 DPMO or 5.5σ are given as comparison chart lines. As depicted, at baseline all results range below industry standards and, thus, are inferior to the overall average. Hence, potential for improvement is correspondingly large.

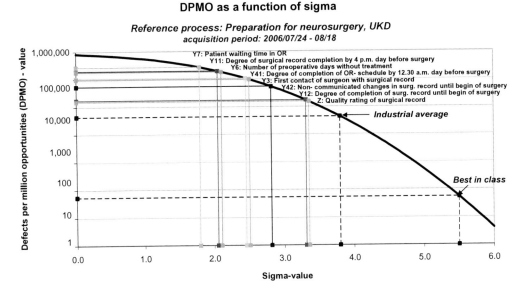

Figure 3. Process performance first measurement phase.

With regard to patient safety the relatively low sigma value of "completion degree of the surgery record on 4 p.m. at surgery- eve "(Y11 = 2.06 σ) represented a major target. From an economic point of view the Sigma value of preoperative number of days without treatment", rather needed improvement (Y6 = 2.11 σ). At this point it must be noted that the very low Sigma values or high DPMO values were not associated with faulty neurosurgery. On the contrary: All surgeries were very well prepared. This result, however, often only was achieved through rework and additional activities in the preparation process for surgery, possibly after work as well as by a certain degree of targeted *ad hoc* action.

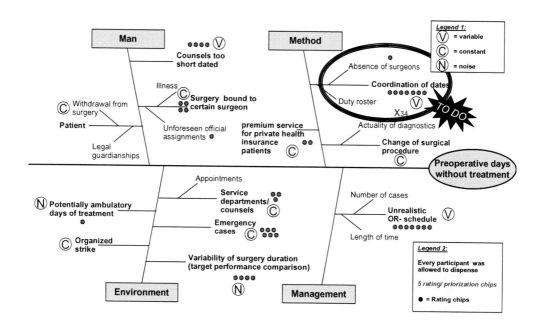

Figure 4. Example Ishikawa diagram

Based on the results of the first measuring phase the present performance of the surgical preparation process was reviewed during the **analysis phase** in detail. The objective was in particular, to uncover main causes of defects/ deviations and, consequently, to derive improvement opportunities. Specifically, in this DMAIC phase, according to the approach in industrial Six Sigma projects the following three steps were accomplished.

1. Identification of potential causes of defects by cause-effect analyses using a series of Ishikawa diagrams (example see Figure 4)
2. Analysis of the current processes and detailed process description using the cross-functional process representation
3. Detection of substantial links between the dependent variables and the independent factors through statistical analysis.

An in depth analysis of the main causes of problems provides the basis for identification and prioritizing improvement measures in a well aimed way. During the **improve-phase** of the Six Sigma project a series of advanced analyses and statistical tests were conducted, e.g., the influence of the chosen OR on the mean waiting time of patients. These tools enabled further trying out and sharpening the impact forecasts as defined at the beginning of the project.

The results of the statistical data analysis had direct impact on the solution finding and selection process. The solution ideas were continuously documented in a MS- Power Point file and were evaluated with regard to their feasibility. Hence a total of 16 ideas could be generated with easy implementability and a high leverage effect with regard to the initial defined CTQs. A diagram representation of the idealized workflow was created subsequently for implementation the solutions, on the basis of the cross functional diagram of the present process, in which all major changes were marked (Figure 5). In order to increase process stability and, thus, the quality of the results, a number of new process steps were defined and inserted into the existing process. The complexity of the surgical preparation process, hence, remained high. Economization was only partially possible, for example by parallelization of sub-processes over time.

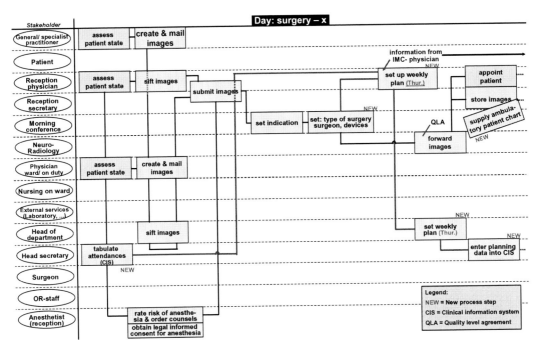

Figure 5. Cross-functional representation of the target process (excerpt)

After the 2-day workshop for the improve phase in October 2006, it took about 5 weeks until the actual process completely could be converted to the target process. For this period a total of 13 individual activities were defined and were implemented gradually.

For example, the following three changes in the target process have been introduced:

1. In addition to the elective care of patients, the emergency procedures are an essential part of operational activities in neurosurgery. Consequently emergency surgeries make up to 10% of all operations, which have to be integrated in the daily elective surgery program because of their urgency. For this reason, a very long-term definitive surgical planning in neurosurgery usually does not make sense. On the other hand, a very short-term surgical planning in individual cases, impairs the timely and thorough surgical preparation. Before the start of the project the OR schedule was planned on the morning of the day before surgery. Within the new ideal workflow a provisional weekly plan is now tabulated and the definitive surgery program is set up two days before the day of surgery. Accordingly, now there is twice as much time for the completion of the surgery preparation and other important pre-operative activities, such as planning the surgery using neuro- navigation, which now can be done on the eve of surgery in peace.

2. Another major change within the optimized process is that the team of outpatient reception now presents the patients in the morning conference. Participants in this

conference are all neurosurgeons, neuroradiologists and case specific physicians from additional departments (pediatrics, ENT, orofacial surgery, radiotherapists, etc.). The case discussion is, thus, decoupled from the stationary admission of patients, which allows a longer-term planning, without unnecessary preoperative inpatient treatment days. At the same time, the available IT planning module for the scheduling of surgeries consistently was used for both, the primary surgical planning as well as for the communication of changes, after appropriate training of employees.

3. The transfer of the patient images required for surgery (X-ray, CT, MRI and angiography images) between the various departments and clinical areas was clearly determined by precise definition of transfer standards and by formulating appropriate operation procedures, to avoid unnecessary search.

The ensuing **control phase** focused on stabilizing the improved preparing for surgery process and to monitor the desired target level. In this context, it had to be verified that the main causes of the problems were eliminated permanently. The results were very satisfactory, so that a comprehensive and meaningful process documentation with visualized target processes and clearly formulated procedural instructions was immediately set up. To achieve a high commitment the latter were thoroughly discussed individually with all stakeholders on the level of suppliers and customers in the Department of Neurosurgery.

After "warming-up" of the fine tuned target process in January / February 2007, a second measurement phase was accomplished. To allow a before and after comparison the same indicators and checklists as in the first measuring phase were used. The survey period again was 20 days of surgery.

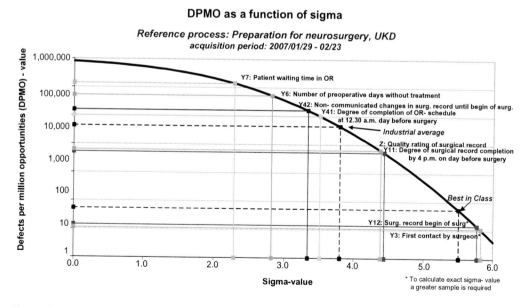

Figure 6. Process performance measurement in the second measurement phase.

Figure 6 represents the DPMO and **sigma results of the second measuring phase** at a glance. In contrast to the results of the baseline measurements in the second measuring phase sigma values of half of the output indicators lay above industry standards, two values are even close to the 6 σ - levels. - All in all, a great project success, which some stakeholders very surprised. The improvement potentials recognized in the measure phase were widely harnessed.

The sigma value of Y11 "completion degree of the surgery record by 4 p.m. on surgeries eve" which is relevant from the patient's viewpoint improved from 2.06 σ to 4.43 σ, corresponding with an advance of the DPMO value by a factor of 170!

Besides the Sigma value, which is relevant in particular for the project leaders and the six sigma black belt, the net benefit is a major target of Six Sigma projects. An internal post calculation confirmed the amount of € 90,000 as assumed in the project charter. For comparison: Experience in industrial companies shows average net benefit ranging from € 50,000 - € 125,000. In calculating the net savings the (cash) cost of the project have to be considered on the one hand. The latter are mainly related to project days / workshops in the clinic. Including preparation and follow-up the total effort amounted 15 project days, spread over 6 months. On the other hand, the financial benefits of the project are to be quantified. It directly or indirectly results from the sigma-value increases. Accordingly, the sigma value of e.g., "number of days without preoperative treatment," rose from 2.11 σ to 2.82 σ representing a DPMO value improvement by a factor of 3. For the commercial board of the University Hospital Dresden solely this detailed figure stands for net savings of about € 25,000 a year, since the preoperative periods dropped by an average of 0.5 days per patient.

CONCLUSION

As the results of this pilot project demonstrate the Six Sigma method is eminently suitable for improving quality of medical processes. All defined **safety relevant quality indicators** were significantly improved by changes in the workflow, as the example of the optimization of preparation for neurosurgery revealed. In detail, the required quality standards of a 100% complete surgical preparation at start of surgery and the required initial contact of the surgeon with the patient/ surgical record on the eve of surgery could be fulfilled within the range of practical zero- defect quality. The cause-effect analysis revealed outstanding importance of these two indicators for patient safety. The more significance has to be attached to the advance of those two key figures into the practical zero- defect range of 6 σ by the implemented changes. Likewise, the degree of completion of the surgical record by 4 p.m. on the eve of surgery and their quality could be improved within the Six Sigma project by a factor of 170 and 16, respectively, at sigma values of 4.43 and 4.38. The other two safety quality indicators "non-communicated changes in the OR- schedule" and the "completeness of the OR- schedule by 12:30 a.m. at the day before surgery" also show an impressive improvement by a factor of 2.8 and 7.7, respectively, corresponding with sigma values of 3.34 and 3.51, even though the industrial average level of quality could not be beaten. In the context of hazards to the health of patients, the latter two figures have an obvious lower weight than the above mentioned four quality indicators.

The focus of the presented Six Sigma project clearly was improvement of patient safety. Accordingly, the six safety related quality indicators showed the highest degree of improvement. At the same time it was, however, impressively shown that a successful quality offensive can, likewise, significantly improve the economic results. In this regard economic "hard facts" as the preoperative length of stay and preventable waiting times in the operating room were favorably affected with an improvement by a factor of 2.9 and 1.8, respectively. In other terms savings of approximately 390 treatment days per year and a reduction in surgical waiting time from an average of 7.6 minutes per surgery could be implemented.

The additional economic benefits of poorly quantifiable effects, such as the reduction of failure costs by avoided human and physical resources required for troubleshooting, future case number increases through enlarged satisfaction of patients, relatives, referring doctors and medical insurances or dropping liability insurance premiums/ avoided liability claims, were not evaluated in the project, however, the latter effects increase the economic advantage in favor of the clinic.

From an economic point of view errors not only rise costs and reduce the financial returns of the company, but can also result in image damage weakening the competitive position of the hospital. With the Six Sigma approach, the hospital management has a successful management approach to its disposal allowing an increase in quality in terms of a workable zero- defect quality with a target of 3.4 DPMO. The quality improvement gained favorably affects the patients' benefits as well as the financial returns of the hospital.

As the present German pilot project showed, the Six Sigma approach also successfully applies for processes in hospitals and other medical facilities. In our experience this methodology is suitable, even for complex clinical processes with a variety of stakeholders. In particular, in processes in which patient safety plays a key role, the objective of achieving a zero- defect quality is reasonable and should definitely be aspirated.

REFERENCES

[1]   Berry R, Murcko AC, Brubaker CE (2002) The Six Sigma Book for Healthcare – Improving outcomes by reducing errors, Chicago

[2]   Günther S., Großekatthöfer J., Sobottka SB, Töpfer A (2008) Weißer Kittel, schwarzer Gürtel - Erstmals SixSigma im deutschen Gesundheitswesen, in: QZ-Qualität und Zuverlässigkeit, Jahrgang 53(2008)4, S. 30-36.

[3]   Institute of Medicine (1999) To err is human: building a safety health system. Washington, DC: National Academy Press

[4]   Pande P, Neumann R, Cavanagh R (2000) The Six Sigma Way: How GE, Motorola, and Other Top Companies Are Honing Their Performance, New York

[5]   Sachverständigenrat für die Konzertierte Aktion im Gesundheitswesen (SVR) (2003) Band I: Finanzierung und Nutzerorientierung. Fassung vom 24.02.2003. www.svr-gesundheit.de/Gutachten/Gutacht03/kurzf-de03.pdf (14.7.2005)

[6]   Harry M, Schroeder R (2006) Six SIGMA: The Breakthrough Management Strategy Revolutionizing the World's Top Corporations, New York

[7]   Sobottka SB, Schackert G (2005a) Proactive clinical risk management in neurosurgery– preliminary experience with employee surveys and an incident reporting system.
       In: Abstracts der 56. Jahrestagung der DGNC, 7.-11.5.2005, Strasbourg

[8]   Sobottka SB, Schackert G (2005b) First experience with a local clinical risk management in neurosurgery – employee surveys and incident reporting system. In: Abstracts of the 13th World Congress of Neurosurgery, Marrakesh 19.-24.6.2005

[9]   Sobottka SB, Schackert G (2006) Employees risk assessment as a basis for preventive clinical risk management in neurosurgery. In: Abstracts der 57. Jahrestagung der DGNC, 11.-14.5.2006, Essen

[10]   Sobottka SB, Reiss G, Eberlein-Gonska M, Töpfer A, Albrecht DM, Schackert G (2007a) Implementation of the Six Sigma Zero Defect Quality Concept in the preparation for neurosurgical procedures. In: Abstracts der 58. Jahrestagung der DGNC,   26.-29.4.2007,   Leipzig,   http://www.egms.de/en/meetings/ dgnc2007/07dgnc364.shtml

[11]   Sobottka SB, Günther S, Großekatthöfer J (2007b) Praktizierte Null-Fehler-Qualität im Krankenhaus durch Six Sigma, in: Klinikmanagement – Der Weg zum wirtschaftlichen wettbewerbsorientierten   Unternehmen,   Schriftlicher   Management-Lehrgang, Euroforum-Verlag 2007, Lektion 8 S. 1-97.

[12]   Thomas EJ, Studdert DM, Burstin HR, Orav EJ, Zeena T, Williams EJ, Howard KM, Weiler PC, Brennan TA (2000) Incidence and types of adverse events and negligent care in Utah and Colorado. Medical Care, 38(3): 261-271

[13]   Töpfer A (2007) Six Sigma als Projektmanagement für höhere Kundenzufriedenheit und bessere Unternehmensergebnisse, in: Töpfer, A. (Hrsg.): Six Sigma: Konzeption und Erfolgsbeispiele für praktizierte Null-Fehler-Qualität, 4. Aufl., Berlin/Heidelberg, S.45–99

[14]   Töpfer A, Großekatthöfer J (2006) Praktizierte Null-Fehler-Qualität durch Six Sigma im   Krankenhaus,   in: Albrecht,   D.   M./Töpfer,   A.   (Eds.):   Erfolgreiches Changemanagement im Krankenhaus: 15-Punkte Sofortprogramm für Kliniken, Heidelberg, S.449–471

In: Dresden Teamwork Concept for Medical...
Editor: Axel R. Heller

ISBN 978-1-60692-307-8
© 2009 Nova Science Publishers, Inc.

Chapter 9

TEAM ORGANIZATION IN THE STROKE NETWORK EAST SAXONY ON THE BASIS OF THE ISO 9001: 2000 QUALITY MANAGEMENT SYSTEM

Georg Gahn

Dresden University Stroke Center, Department of Neurology
University Hospital Carl Gustav Carus, University of Technology, Dresden, Germany

ABSTRACT

Background: East Saxony is a rural area with approx. 1,600,000 citizens. In the capital Dresden with approx. 500,000 citizens two stroke units are located. Stroke patients outside Dresden are usually treated in general hospitals without stroke expertise. We developed a model for widespread stroke care throughout East- Saxony based on a cooperative network between a comprehensive stroke center (CSC) and several affiliated general hospitals (Stroke-East-Saxony Network - SOS-NET). We applied the quality management (QM-)system ISO 9001:2000 as the basis for quality assurance.

Methods: We attempted to certify interdisciplinary stroke care at CSC according to the requirements of the German Stroke Association and to ISO 9001:2000 standard. The quality standards of CSC are transferred to affiliated hospitals and established by on site training sessions. Structural, process and result quality are assured by regular audits. Acute stroke therapy in the affiliated hospitals is guided through a video conference.

Results: In June 2007, CSC was certified. So far, five satellite hospitals were approved by CSC as cooperating partners in stroke care covering approx. 500,000 citizens outside Dresden. So far, 116 patients were presented for acute stroke treatment via video conference. Negotiations for cooperation are underway with 5 more hospitals

Conclusion: Acute stroke therapy in rural areas appears to be feasible on a high quality level if applying a certified QM-system in combination with a video conference system.

ABBREVIATIONS

ADSR = German Stroke Registers Study Group
CSC = Comprehensive Stroke Center
DUSC = Dresden University Stroke Center
ISO = International Organization for Standardization
JCAHO = Joint Commission on Accreditation of Health Organizations
PSC = Primary Stroke Center
QM = Quality Management
SOP = Standard Operational Procedure
SOS-NET = Stroke East Saxony Network

INTRODUCTION

Since the onset and establishment of stroke units, acute stroke management has been dramatically changed with increasing numbers of patients being treated with t-PA thrombolysis, the only approved drug therapy for acute ischemic stroke [1]. Also medical aspects of acute stroke care have been shown to improve stroke patients´ outcome [2]. Both, thrombolysis and the specialized medical stroke care are provided by stroke units. Some western countries have managed to provide acute stroke care by stroke units to almost all regional residents, most have not [3].

Recently, several attempts have been made to provide acute stroke care via telemedicine to patients in rural areas located far away from hospitals with expertise in stroke care [4-10]. Whether telemedicine represents the appropriate tool for treating acute stroke patients outside stroke units is discussed controversially. Cerebral ischemia represents a complex pathophysiological and organizational situation requiring highly specialized, multidisciplinary, and multiprofessional management [11]. Telemedicine could be restricted to be a helpful supportive technique in the acute stroke setting guiding the decision towards or against t-PA therapy. However, the concomitant conservative stroke care remains an equally important issue which needs to be addressed consequently and which can not be provided by telemedicine.

Dedicated stroke care is hard and expensive to establish. Therefore many countries require quality standards to be fulfilled by certified stroke centers [12-17]. In the U.S., the Joint Commission on Accreditation of Health Organizations (JCAHO) offers a widely accepted quality management (QM-) system. Recently a special program has been established focusing on so called "primary stroke centers" (PSC) [18]. In the US, members of the Brain Attack Coalition have published recommendations for establishment of comprehensive stroke centers (CSC) capable of delivering the full spectrum of care to seriously ill patients with stroke and cerebrovascular diseases [19]. Currently efforts are made to certify CSCs according to an independent QM-system, since self-certification is likely to lead to a significant overestimation of a hospital's compliance with published recommendations suggesting outside independent evaluations of hospitals as stroke centers [20]. In Europe outside evaluation of PSCs or CSCs by certified QM-systems is still pending [12].

We challenge that a CSC should provide excellent multidisciplinary stroke care for its own urban residents and should be controlled by an independent and certified QM-system. A

CSC should also establish wide spread high level stroke care in the surrounding rural areas applying an appropriate quality assurance system.

METHODS

We established SOS-NET (Stroke East-Saxony-Network – *"East" translates in German "Ost"*) applying four steps:

1. Establishment of an independent QM-system for stroke care at CSC entitled "Dresden University Stroke Center" (DUSC) according to the internationally accepted European standardized QM-system, the International Organization for Standardization (ISO) 9001:2000 [21].
2. Transfer and control of our quality standards to general hospitals located outside the city borders and willing to cooperate as affiliated hospitals in acute stroke care as members of the SOS-NET.
3. Establishment of a video conference systems to guide acute stroke therapy in affiliated hospitals by DUSC.

Ad 1.) The ISO 9001:2000 is an European QM-system addressing multiple aspects of quality assurance [21]. In brief, nearly all institutional activities are divided into supportive, core, and managing processes [22]. Supportive processes refer to the management of facilities, core processes to the patient care itself and management processes mainly to management of human recourses. All processes participating in acute stroke care are subjects to a continuous improvement process, a so called P-D-C-A (plan-do-check-act) cycle [23]. An external ISO 9001:2000 audit with re-evaluation of DUSC is regularly done in yearly intervals. Our strategic goal is to establish the ISO 9001:2000 quality standard for stroke care throughout all departments participating in acute stroke care, e.g., neurology, neurosurgery, neuroradiology, cardiology, vascular surgery, anesthesiology, and clinical chemistry.

Ad 2.) The cooperating hospitals all signed a written contract containing detailed quality standards of stroke care. These quality standards contain criteria about those patients to be presented by videoconference, those patients to be transferred to CSC, detailed requirements for a stroke clinical pathway (process quality) and for structural resources dedicated to stroke care. The requirements are in concordance to those required for PSCs in Europe [12]. The only difference is the missing permanent availability (24 hours/7days) of a neurologist. The cooperating hospitals are all checked once a year during an on site visit performed by specially trained DUSC auditors (according to ISO 9001:2000 standards).

Ad 3.) All cooperating stroke hospitals are equipped with a videoconference system (Meytec™, Berlin, Germany) permitting real-time physical examination of stroke patients in the emergency room (see Figure 1) [24;25]. Additionally, neuroimaging data can be transferred in DICOM format from the regional hospital to a central SOS-NET server [26]. This server can be accessed by DUSC to view neuroimaging data. Data transferred during videoconference are secured by a VPN tunneling. Inspection of the patient by videoconference is possible from two stationary PCs located on the stroke unit and on the intensive care unit of DUSC as well as from two portable notebooks using UMTS-connection for wireless data transfer. The portable variant permits home work during night shift for those employees working as tele-consultants. All tele-consultants are neurologist and have been trained at least for one year on our stroke unit, one year on our neurological intensive care unit, three months on a cardiological intensive care unit, and two months in our neurovascular ultrasound laboratory. Additionally they received special training in stroke CT-reading. Every three months a quality care meeting between the tele-consultants takes place, as well as an advisory board meeting of DUSC members with all cooperating SOS-NET partners.

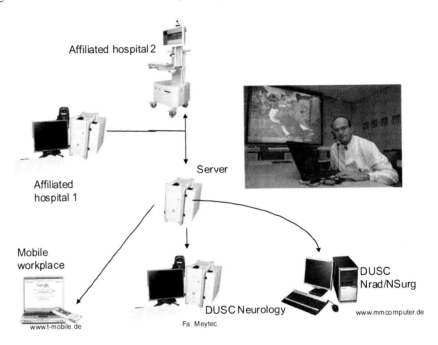

Figure 1. Technological equipment used for teleconferences.

The tele-consultation is initiated by the on call physician in the affiliated hospital calling an exclusive "SOS-NET cellular phone number" of the tele-consultant. The tele-consultant then contacts the cooperating hospital via videoconference. In case of technical problems with the videoconference system, conversation via SOS-NET cellular phone still provides a rescue solution [27].

The tele-consultation follows a structured protocol beginning with a brief anamnesis (personal data, onset of symptoms), followed by a physical examination according to the National Institutes of Health Stroke Scale (NIHSS) [28], an inspection of the computed tomography with grading the area of ischemia according to the ASPECTS (Alberta Stroke Program CT Score) [29], a detailed checklist containing exclusion criteria against thrombolysis, and a concluding assessment and therapeutic plan. For certain aspects of the NIHSS help by a nurse or physician maybe requested during tele consultation.

The remote medical personnel (physicians and nurses) is trained at the beginning of the cooperation and once a year in performing NIHSS assessment following the suggestions of Lyden et al. [30]. Apart of that twice a year stroke education is offered at DUSC to all SOS-NET participants and once a year at the affiliated hospitals by members of DUSC. Also in-house visits for medical personnel at DUSC are offered to all SOS-NET participants.

Technical equipment is financed by the Saxony Ministry of Social Care, Family and Health. Maintenance costs are currently paid by the SOS-NET partners. Negotiations with health care companies to finance maintenance costs are currently underway.

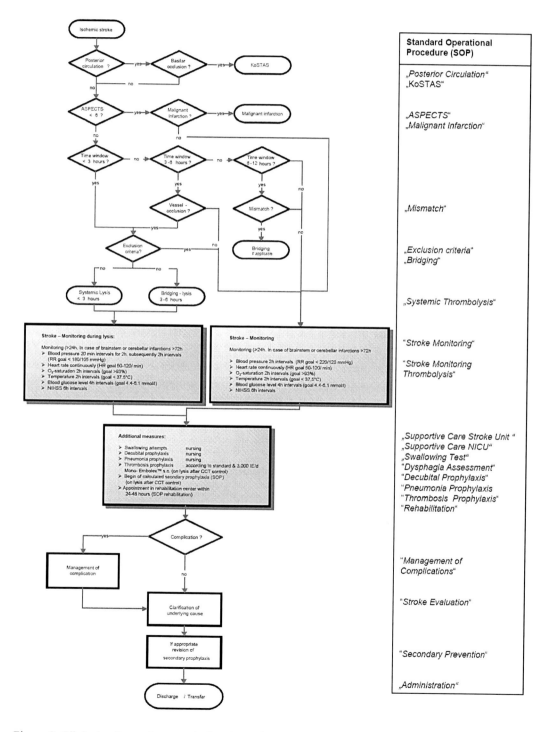

Figure 2. Clinical pathway for acute ischemic stroke.

For assessment of outcome quality we use a modified stroke questionnaire of the German Stroke Registers Study Group (ADSR) [31]. Briefly, the ADSR questionnaire contains information about the acute stroke phase (e.g., onset to treatment time, door-to needle time, NIHSS on admission) as well as information about the hospital course (e.g., final diagnosis, modified Rankin scale at discharge, risk factors, reason for cerebral ischemia, initiation of therapy). We added items regarding tele consultation and outcome after three months (modified Rankin scale, medical therapy of risk factors). Questionnaires are machine readable, data are downloaded in a SPSS-database. All patients treated in the SOS-NET are contacted by telephone interview three months after stroke onset. Primary outcome data are death and disabling stroke defined as a modified Ranking scale ≥3. Secondary outcome data are continuation of secondary prevention medication for stroke risk factors.

RESULTS

Certification of DUSC took place in June 2007 and was done both by the German Stroke Association and according to ISO 9001:2000 QM-system (LG Intercert, Erlangen, Germany). In a first step the stroke unit and the neurological intensive care unit of DUSC analyzed its own structural, process and outcome quality exposing the stroke unit and intensive care unit to a continuous improvement process. As core processes we chose ischemic and hemorrhagic stroke, subarachnoid hemorrhage, carotid artery stenosis, and cerebral venous thrombosis: We considered these diseases to represent the major categories of stroke in our institution. SOPs and clinical pathways were generated for all these core processes in an interdisciplinary and multiprofessional approach spanning the time frame from notification by emergency service over hospital admission to discharge (see Figure 2). Affiliated departments like neurosurgery, neuroradiology, cardiology, clinical chemistry, vascular surgery, and speech therapy were first connected by quality assurance contracts. Supportive, core, and management processes are all collected in a so called management handbook, being available online throughout the hospital.

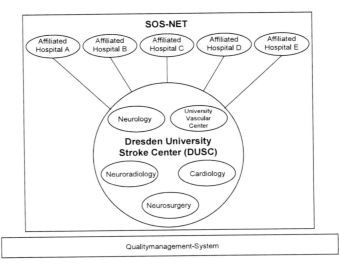

Figure 3. Structure of SOS-NET and DUSC.

The QM-system is controlled by a core group meeting taking place every week during preparation for certification and twice a months afterwards. All meeting results and all planned action is documented in standardized protocols and offered to all employees of the department via intranet. Twice a year the director of DUSC is supposed to present perform-ance data of DUSC and SOS-NET to a board of directors consisting of the medical and the economical CEOs of the hospital, the Dean of the medical faculty, and the head of the hospi-tals´ QM-department. Structure of DUSC is outlined by rules of procedures signed by the board of directors (see Figure 3).

The two first SOS-NET affiliated hospitals were audited in June 2007 by DUSC for structural and process quality in stroke care. The third one followed February 2008, the fourth one in May 2008, the fifth one in June 2008. These five hospitals cover a region of approx. 100 km in diameter around Dresden with approx. 500.000 citizens (see Figure 4). DUSC per-formed two local training sessions in all SOS-NET affiliated hospitals before initiation of cooperation and offered two central stroke lectures for SOS-NET affiliated hospitals. Tele-consultations started July first 2007. So far 116 consultations took place. Five more hospitals are in negotiations for SOS-NET affiliation.

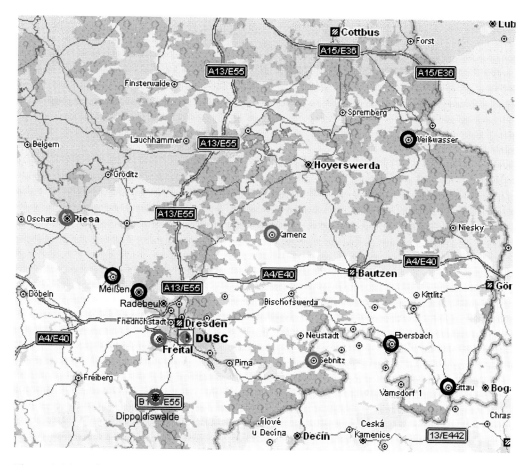

Figure 4. Map of East Saxony (north direction top of map; right margin Polish |——25 km——| Republic; south border Czech Republic) showing Dresden University Stroke Center (DUSC) and the affiliated hospitals in the SOS-NET (pink circles: hospitals cooperating already in daily routine, black circles: hospitals under negotiations).

CONCLUSIONS

We present an ambitious project to establish widespread high quality acute stroke care in a rural area to patients otherwise not having access to this type of care because of long distances to stroke units.

We chose the ISO 9001:2000 quality standard since we consider the structure of this system to be easily adjustable to the health care system. The JCAHO provides a special program for dedicated stroke centers but has less emphasis on a continuous improvement process which appears to be most valuable to us. On the other hand the JCAHO criteria for PSC are already part of national US guidelines [32] which is not the case for the ISO QM-system in Europe.

A matter of debate represents the patients´ consent into the consultation via tele-conference. In case of a wake patient the patient may be asked to sign or to consent in the presence of a witness. In case of inability to understand or to consent, the emergency situation of acute stroke does not offer an alternative to therapy with t-PA, the only licensed drug for acute stroke therapy. t-PA therapy could only be withheld in presence of appropriate advance directives.

Another legal uncertainty represents the situation of treating a patient via teleconference. Even though data transfer is secured by a VPN tunneling, treating a patient is a personal act and not an act that can be provided through television [33]. In SOS-NET, responsibility for patients´ treatment remains in the affiliated hospitals by contract. However, current legislation may also contribute a partial responsibility to the tele-consultant who guides the therapy with his expertise [33].

Certainly tele-consultation for acute stroke therapy represents a spectacular tool for patient management which can be easily used as a marketing initiative by competing hospitals. It has been shown by others that tele-consultation and transfer of quality standards to the network partners improve patients´ outcome and reduces financial burdens of the health care system [34;35]. Therefore tele-consultation appears to be an attractive extension to the hospitals´ portfolios. Nevertheless stroke care is rather not limited to application of t-PA but requires highly trained and experienced personnel to achieve optimal process and outcome quality. General hospitals applying thrombolysis to acute stroke patients in the context of a tele-consultation should also provide appropriate stroke care apart of thrombolysis. This issue gains importance in a setting, when highly specialized medical expertise is only punctually applied to patients by video conference systems but continuous patient care is far out of range of the specialists and hardly controllable. We consider our QM-model of establishing a continuous quality improvement process in the affiliated hospitals as a prerequisite for high quality stroke care beyond t-PA application.

The economical perspective provides a win-win situation to all participants. The center earns financial benefit by selling the tele-consultations to the affiliated hospitals. Stroke patients, who are potential candidates for interventions or therapeutic studies can be very early directed to the center providing new chances for interventions or clinical studies. The affiliated hospitals can admit and treat patients in a way they are not able to without support by external stroke specialists. Finally the health care providers save money through better patients´ outcome and lowering the burden of social costs.

In conclusion, we suggest to widespread acute stroke care to rural areas by establishing CSCs with connected networks of affiliated tele-stroke hospitals on the basis of an independent and certified QM-system such as the ISO 9001:2000.

REFERENCES

[1]   Hacke W, Donnan G, Fieschi C, Kaste M, von Kummer R, Broderick JP, et al. Association of outcome with early stroke treatment: pooled analysis of ATLANTIS, ECASS, and NINDS rt-PA stroke trials. Lancet 2004 Mar 6;363(9411):768-74.

[2]   Candelise L, Gattinoni M, Bersano A, Micieli G, Sterzi R, Morabito A. Stroke-unit care for acute stroke patients: an observational follow-up study. Lancet 2007 Jan 27;369(9558):299-305.

[3]   Leys D, Ringelstein EB, Kaste M, Hacke W. Facilities available in European hospitals treating stroke patients. Stroke 2007 Nov;38(11):2985-91.

[4]   Audebert HJ, Schenkel J, Heuschmann PU, Bogdahn U, Haberl RL. Effects of the implementation of a telemedical stroke network: the Telemedic Pilot Project for Integrative Stroke Care (TEMPiS) in Bavaria, Germany. Lancet Neurol 2006 Sep;5(9):742-8.

[5]   Choi JY, Porche NA, Albright KC, Khaja AM, Ho VS, Grotta JC. Using telemedicine to facilitate thrombolytic therapy for patients with acute stroke. Jt Comm J Qual Patient Saf 2006 Apr;32(4):199-205.

[6]   Waite K, Silver F, Jaigobin C, Black S, Lee L, Murray B, et al. Telestroke: a multi-site, emergency-based telemedicine service in Ontario. J Telemed Telecare 2006;12(3):141-5.

[7]   Hess DC, Wang S, Gross H, Nichols FT, Hall CE, Adams RJ. Telestroke: extending stroke expertise into underserved areas. Lancet Neurol 2006 Mar;5(3):275-8.

[8]   Handschu R, Littmann R, Reulbach U, Gaul C, Heckmann JG, Neundorfer B, et al. Telemedicine in emergency evaluation of acute stroke: interrater agreement in remote video examination with a novel multimedia system. Stroke 2003 Dec;34(12):2842-6.

[9]   Wiborg A, Widder B. Teleneurology to improve stroke care in rural areas: The Telemedicine in Stroke in Swabia (TESS) Project. Stroke 2003 Dec;34(12):2951-6.

[10] Shafqat S, Kvedar JC, Guanci MM, Chang Y, Schwamm LH. Role for telemedicine in acute stroke. Feasibility and reliability of remote administration of the NIH stroke scale. Stroke 1999 Oct;30(10):2141-5.

[11] Leys D, Ringelstein EB, Kaste M, Hacke W. Facilities available in European hospitals treating stroke patients. Stroke 2007 Nov;38(11):2985-91.

[12] Leys D, Ringelstein EB, Kaste M, Hacke W. The main components of stroke unit care: results of a European expert survey. Cerebrovasc Dis 2007;23(5-6):344-52.

[13] Czlonkowska A, Sarzynska-Dlugosz I, Niewada M, Kobayashi A. Eligibility of stroke units in Poland for administration of intravenous thrombolysis. Eur J Neurol 2006 Mar;13(3):220-4.

[14] Organised inpatient (stroke unit) care for stroke. Cochrane Database Syst Rev 2007;(4):CD000197.

[15] Hack W, Kaste M, Bogousslavsky J, Brainin M, Chamorro A, Lees K, et al. European Stroke Initiative Recommendations for Stroke Management-update 2003. Cerebrovasc Dis 2003;16(4):311-37.

[16] Adams R, Acker J, Alberts M, Andrews L, Atkinson R, Fenelon K, et al. Recommendations for improving the quality of care through stroke centers and systems: an examination of stroke center identification options: multidisciplinary consensus recommendations from the Advisory Working Group on Stroke Center Identification Options of the American Stroke Association. Stroke 2002 Jan;33(1):e1-e7.

[17] Park S, Schwamm LH. Organizing regional stroke systems of care. Curr Opin Neurol 2008 Feb;21(1):43-55.

[18] Primary Stroke Center Certification. http://www.jointcommission.org/ CertificationPrograms/PrimaryStrokeCenters/. 25-5-2008. Ref Type: Internet Communication

[19] Alberts MJ, Latchaw RE, Selman WR, Shephard T, Hadley MN, Brass LM, et al. Recommendations for comprehensive stroke centers: a consensus statement from the Brain Attack Coalition. Stroke 2005 Jul;36(7):1597-616.

[20] Kidwell CS, Shephard T, Tonn S, Lawyer B, Murdock M, Koroshetz W, et al. Establishment of primary stroke centers: A survey of physician attitudes and hospital resources. Neurology 2003 May 13;60(9):1452-6.

[21] Carson BE. ISO 9001:2000---A New Paradigm for Healthcare. ASQ Quality Press; 2004.

[22] Beholz S, Koch C, Konertz W. Quality management system of a university cardiac surgery department according to DIN EN ISO 9001 : 2000. Thorac Cardiovasc Surg 2003 Jun;51(3):167-73.

[23] Van Scyoc K. Process safety improvement--Quality and target zero. Journal of Hazardous MaterialsIn Press, Corrected Proof.

[24] Shafqat S, Kvedar JC, Guanci MM, Chang Y, Schwamm LH. Role for telemedicine in acute stroke. Feasibility and reliability of remote administration of the NIH stroke scale. Stroke 1999 Oct;30(10):2141-5.

[25] Wang S, Lee SB, Pardue C, Ramsingh D, Waller J, Gross H, et al. Remote evaluation of acute ischemic stroke: reliability of National Institutes of Health Stroke Scale via telestroke. Stroke 2003 Oct;34(10):e188-e191.

[26] Johnston KC, Worrall BB. Teleradiology Assessment of Computerized Tomographs Online Reliability Study (TRACTORS) for acute stroke evaluation. Telemed J E Health 2003;9(3):227-33.

[27] Frey JL, Jahnke HK, Goslar PW, Partovi S, Flaster MS. tPA by telephone: extending the benefits of a comprehensive stroke center. Neurology 2005 Jan 11;64(1):154-6.

[28] Shafqat S, Kvedar JC, Guanci MM, Chang Y, Schwamm LH. Role for Telemedicine in Acute Stroke : Feasibility and Reliability of Remote Administration of the NIH Stroke Scale. Stroke 1999 Oct 1;30(10):2141-5.

[29] Barber PA, Demchuk AM, Zhang J, Buchan AM. Validity and reliability of a quantitative computed tomography score in predicting outcome of hyperacute stroke before thrombolytic therapy. ASPECTS Study Group. Alberta Stroke Programme Early CT Score. Lancet 2000 May 13;355(9216):1670-4.

[30] Lyden P, Brott T, Tilley B, Welch KM, Mascha EJ, Levine S, et al. Improved reliability of the NIH Stroke Scale using video training. NINDS TPA Stroke Study Group. Stroke 1994 Nov;25(11):2220-6.

[31] Heuschmann PU, Biegler MK, Busse O, Elsner S, Grau A, Hasenbein U, et al. Development and Implementation of Evidence-Based Indicators for Measuring Quality of Acute Stroke Care: The Quality Indicator Board of the German Stroke Registers Study Group (ADSR). Stroke 2006 Oct 1;37(10):2573-51.

[32] Adams HP, Jr., del Zoppo G, Alberts MJ, Bhatt DL, Brass L, Furlan A, et al. Guidelines for the Early Management of Adults With Ischemic Stroke: A Guideline From the American Heart Association/ American Stroke Association Stroke Council, Clinical Cardiology Council, Cardiovascular Radiology and Intervention Council, and the Atherosclerotic Peripheral Vascular Disease and Quality of Care Outcomes in Research Interdisciplinary Working Groups: The American Academy of Neurology affirms the value of this guideline as an educational tool for neurologists. Stroke 2007 May 1;38(5):1655-711.

[33] Stanberry B. Legal and ethical aspects of telemedicine. J Telemed Telecare 2006;12(4):166-75.

[34] Schwab S, Vatankhah B, Kukla C, Hauchwitz M, Bogdahn U, Furst A, et al. Long-term outcome after thrombolysis in telemedical stroke care. Neurology 2007 Aug 28;69(9):898-903.

[35] Audebert HJ, Schenkel J, Heuschmann PU, Bogdahn U, Haberl RL. Effects of the implementation of a telemedical stroke network: the Telemedic Pilot Project for Integrative Stroke Care (TEMPiS) in Bavaria, Germany. Lancet Neurol 2006 Sep;5(9):742-8.

In: Dresden Teamwork Concept for Medical…
Editor: Axel R. Heller

ISBN 978-1-60692-307-8
© 2009 Nova Science Publishers, Inc.

Chapter 10

COMMUNICATION AND TEAM MANAGEMENT IN DISASTER MEDICINE

Axel R. Heller and Michael P. Müller

Department of Anesthesiology & Critical Care Medicine,
University Hospital Carl Gustav Carus, University of Technology, Dresden, Germany

ABSTRACT

Multidisciplinary communication activities during mass casualty incidents are double edged because they must be subordinated under the major goal of mental model alignment of all participants to implement a joint strategy under time pressure. In particular during the early stages of a mass casualty incident tactical relevant information has to be filtered from a flood of data while organizational structure of emergency support is only slowly growing up. Excessive communication activities on a limited bandwidth reduce the signal/noise ratio and, hence, impede transmission of relevant information.

Implementing organizational structure and subsidiary leadership within subunits facilitate the accomplishment of the primary goals by reducing tactical communication to a minimum. Medical Emergency Tags in this regard are a simple but valuable communication tool to give comprehensive information to the relevant decision makers, also allowing tracking patients´ condition and tracing their final destination.

As in modern business management the organizational structure must follow the process which itself is determined by strategy. To assure proper implementation of strategy the communication structure has lastly to emulate the chain of command, and, by this means limits communication to those forces who must exchange information with each other. Further a unified management culture across all Emergency management organizations and agencies by a joint leadership manual e.g., DV100 focusing on the establishing a functional global organization facilitates timely implementation.

ABBREVIATIONS

CCP Casualty collection point; **CCT** Command & Communication Truck; **DMAT** Disaster Medical Assistance Team (**-M**) Medical; (**-G**) Guardianship; (**-S**) Supply; **EMS** Emergency Medical Service; **EOC** Emergency Operations Center; **FCCSP** Fundamental Crit. Care Support Physician; **FD** Fire Department; **FEMA** Federal Emergency Management Agencies; **GP** General Practitioner; **HEICS** Hospital Emergency Incident Command System; **IC** Incident Command; **MCI** Mass Casualty Incident; **METTAG** Medical Emergency Triage Tag; **PD** Police Department; **PPE** Personal protective equipment; **ROC** Regular Operations Command; **TA** Transportation Area

INTRODUCTION

The joint Saxon law on fire defense, emergency services and disaster defense (SächsBRKG) issued in 2004, is one of the latest rescue service laws in Germany, having received major impetus by the experiences of Elbe floods 2002 in terms of inter-cooperation and communication between official agencies and organizations [1;2]. In line with its cross-organizational authority, it is also known as "blue light law." In Section 2, Paragraph 3 it defines a disaster as:

... An incident, threatening or damaging life, health, the supply of the population with essential goods and services, the environment or substantial property in such extraordinary manner that assistance and protection can only be granted if the competent authorities and agencies, organizations and workforces collaborate under the unified leadership of a civil protection authority.

The latter defined necessity not only applies to mass casualty incidents (MCI) and disasters, but also to scenarios below the disaster threshold [3-6]. Disasters or major hazard situations are characterized by a lack or a destruction of infrastructure and the needs of multiple victims overwhelm medical services' capacity of care [7-9]. The usual individual maximum care under these circumstances can not be guaranteed. Consequently, the allocation of resources in the early stages always has to be prioritized considering efficiency [8-11]. In this regard the need of wide-ranging assistance strongly depends on the local Emergency Medical Service (EMS) structure. So, in rural areas an accident with five seriously injured persons might have the impact of a MCI due to lower resource density. Regardless of the latter, operations command of conventional large damage scenarios is prepared to utilize the initially quantitatively limited resources in such a way that individual medical care, being the normal emergency services case is restored as quickly as possible [11;12].

STRATEGY → PROCESS → ORGANIZATIONAL STRUCTURE → COMMUNICATION STRUCTURE

Key points of medical disaster missions are first defining treatment and transport priorities (triage), second the concentration of patients and few resources in one place as well as buffering low priority patients by time [5].

Table 1: MCI Quick reference: "Communication tasks" of first arriving/ Chief FCCS Physician

1. [] Report arrival on scene to ROC
2. [] Contact with first arriving service/ earliest FCCS/ EMS Chief / FD Chief (+ radio accessibility)
3. [] Self-protection of forces (PPE), dynamics of damage development
4. [] Delegations/ rough structuring
5. [] Situation assessment (preliminary definition of internal/ external perimeter sections)
   [] Casualty collection points [] / prevailing wind!/ Ready areas for approaching forces []
6. [] Initial rough triage with short documentary (streak list)
   Numbers with colored marker/ color tape to victims forehead.
7. [] Feedback to ROC/ targeted request for additional forces,
   Motor vehicle approach order, request 2 DMAT-M, 1 DMAT-G, 1 DMAT-S,
   Alternate radio channel/ municipal bus
8. [] Coordination with chiefs FD/ PD/ EMS (link command posts/ setup local command center/ IC, secure communications) Dynamics? Hazards?
9. [] Spatial structure of the scene (definitive determination of item 5 []) setup provisional CCP with EMS material/staff. (CCT or related to location, size, and type of incident preplanned location (EOC) far removed from incident)
10. [] Organizational structure of operations area / assign resources to tactical level areas, provide tactical objectives for divisions & groups on scene
11. [] Second and definite triaging and tagging of casualties (METTAGS)
12. [] Second report to ROC including general injury patterns,
    HEICS → major incident standby
13. [] Provide tactical and staffing objectives for second wave forces (TA chief)
14. [] Separate green tagged casualties physically (minor treatment/ bus) and secure medical support (any physician (GP), ambulance car, 2m FM-radio)
15. [] Delegation of therapeutic measures for all tagging categories in definite CCPs
16. [] Set transport priority for the red and yellow tagged
17. [] Documentation of individual destination hospitals and feedback to ROC. (also possible by EMS with regard to authorization by CP-FCCS)
18. [] Food and associated supplies, rehabilitation of personnel
19. [] Set destinations for further transports/ documentation []
20. [] Media Information / coordination with IC/ PD/ FD
21. [] Debriefing

Examples of different transport priorities are: Upper extremity fracture (minimal therapy), stable abdominal wounds (delayed therapy) and unstable pneumothorax (immediate treatment, then high transport priority). To enforce this strategy as soon as the first arriving forces have to begin with the set up of a situation adapted infrastructure (Table 1).

Shortcomings during the initial phase are, if at all, hard to overcome in the forthcoming course. These tactical goals together with the earlier mentioned definition of a disaster demand for an intact vertical chain of communication within any organization to secure completion of tasks such as fire fighting, medical, or technical assistance, etc.. At the same time, however, it must be ensured that tasks are horizontally coordinated (across organizations) in a target or strategy oriented manner and mutual interdisciplinary advisory is practiced, as postulated in modern management [13;14].

This implies that the communication (-infra-) structure emulates the chain of command. In this regard it is crucial that the coordination of targets between the organizations is accomplished on the same level of command, controlling the whole operational area of the respective services [15-17] and sharing one mental model of both, the situation and the response strategy [18]. Independent direct interaction of operational forces of different professional services may impact the overall strategy harmful, as illustrated in the following example.

As part of the evacuation operation of a clinic during the Elbe floods in 2002 (see chapter 11) EMS vehicles had a patient pick-up mission from the outpatient reception of a certain hospital. The arriving EMS cars were redirected by doctors of other hospital units to *"their"* buildings on the site, loaded the patients from these doctors (in opposition to global strategy) and left the hot zone with their patients. From the perspective of the third level Emergency Operations Command (EOC) evacuation seemed to run on schedule because they sent vehicles which loaded and departed. The operational control center within the hospital, however, waited in vain for EMS until the issue was clear. Would the command structure have been emulated by the communication structure and the coordination would have taken place on operational section level, misleading communication with the result of uncoordinated transports, not according to priority could have been avoided.

INTEGRATION OF THE AVAILABLE COMMUNICATION TECHNOLOGY INTO THE COMMUNICATION PHILOSOPHY

For the communication between EMS, Federal Emergency Management Agencies (FEMA) and organizations with public security tasks (FD/ PD) FM radio channels in the 4m- and the 2m band are available in Germany. In this regard the 4m devices serve for communication between vehicles and the control center in a range of 20-30 km. Through the distribution of relay stations, radio coverage of a district (radio traffic area) can be realized. In each radio traffic area besides the regular operations channel one to two additional 4m channels per specialist service are available.

In large scale incidents early uncoupling of routine operations from the scene is advisable, to relocate the incident communication to an additional FM-channel being managed by a separate control center dispatcher. If using a mobile operational control center (Command truck/ unified command), a decentralized on scene leadership via the alternate 4m-channels can be implemented. Command communication within the incident perimeter by the unified command and respective tactical branches is accomplished by the use of portable 2m FM radios, ranging 100m to 2km depending on terrain and buildings.

The use of 2m FM radio is assigned by the Incident Command who separates the situation in communication groups through the channel assignment. Due to the limitation of the usual 2m analog devices in use with up to ten channels, the number of sharable channels across the participating organizations is three to four. Depending on the extent of the situation, the number of assigned geographic, technical and organizational sections, and the separate (horizontal) communicating levels of the hierarchy, this bandwidth is undersupplied. Shared use of channels by different professional services hampers the targeted trouble-free communication and makes sense at most on a command "gold" channel.

The primary objective in the implementation of a communication structure is the proper communication between such forces, units or agencies which *must* exchange information with each other to assure the smooth deployment of mission. Furthermore, if the communication structure is designed in a way to emulate the desired command structure, units or forces being not directly linked within hierarchy may not even get in touch with each other. By this means adherence to hierarchical command and reporting chains is enforced.

Common Communication Problems

Basically, telecommunication problems arise from missing or failing technology or bandwidth (objective lack of communication channels), quantitative overload of existing technology (relative lack of communication channels) and lack of effectiveness of communication itself.

If the narrow bandwidth in the analog radio system is blocked with low information content, communication activity strongly increases, especially because information, resulting measure orders, and respective controls goad each other in the sense of a back coupling. As a consequence, the transmission of important information arises to a question of chance until all communications collapse. This is particularly true for the 2m-FM radio, but during peak times, likewise, applies for the 4m band.

Experience shows that the alternative use of cellular phones in such situations is also limited because many forces and in particular third parties occupy lines and, thus, overload the network (if available at all). In the US the ACCOLC procedure (ACCess Overload Control for cellular radio telephones) shuts down the cellular phone network to a predefined user group of forces on request of the police control center [19]. In Germany the joint manual of public security agencies (DV 100) also provides such possibility. Whether or not these additional communication opportunities are of tactical value, is questionable (actuality of authorization lists, shortly required additional users, etc.). In smaller incidents, the network is not overstrained, so that a network shut down would not be justified. Conversely, own experiences in Elbe flood in 2002 show that mobile connections of executive persons are so busy that communication, is not actually facilitated [20]. Furthermore battery capacity may also be limiting.

Distinct organizations currently evaluate the on scene benefits of industry- standard DECT phones. Standards do, accordingly, do neither exist within nor across organizations. Moreover, the disruptive influence of DECT to electronic medical products e.g., patient monitors has to be considered. Future must show in how far wireless local area network (WLAN) technology or universal mobile telecommunication systems (UMTS) in combination with tabletop PCs will facilitate management on scene. Using such technology additional features besides others could be automated data/ status interchange also with the world wide web to enable on-line visualization of the scene by tactical maps on the level of incident command without the need of additional vertical verbal communication.

Medical Emergency Triage Tags (Mettags) as a Communication Medium

In addition to patient lists on the level of operations sections minimum records of the patients' condition must be currently available. Especially during the first information gathering phase organized by the regular EMS repeated investigations of patients (an average of 90 seconds per patient is available) must be avoided at all costs, to allow a definite determination and request of further needs as early as possible, and to start individually prioritized patient care afterwards.

Table 2: Tagging categories (Germany) [8;9]

Category	Definition	Transport	Code
I	Vital threat → Immediate treatment	Immediate after treatment	red
II	Severely injured/ ill without vital threat → delayed treatment	Expedited	yellow
III	Lightly injured/ ill → Minor treatment/ Consolidated care	As soon as possible	green
IV	Observant treatment when medical needs overwhelm capabilities / Dead people	Low priority	blue

After individual examination by a FCCS provider, the triage category of the individual patient (table 2) will be made visible at first glance by the color codes of the METTAG. In a simplified version, the color marking of the patients with their triage category on the forehead with waterproof marker or tape (red: code red, white: others) turned out to be efficient [3]. The current findings and treatments are noted on the METTAGs, allowing tracking of the individual patient's condition. Two copies of the original, which remains with the patient return to the operational command (tracing service), one by the transportation chief (departure) and the other one by the target clinic (arrivals) in order to fully document the patients whereabouts. In a mass casualty incident an average of approximately 20% victims are red and yellow code, respectively, 40% are tagged green and 10% blue. Further 10% casualties must be assumed primarily dead [3].

ESTABLISHMENT OF A COMMAND AND COMMUNICATION STRUCTURE FOR LARGE SCALE INCIDENTS

In the early stages of a major incident there will be a significant flow of information to the few even temporary executives, exceeding the threshold of processing and response capacity by far [21]. Personal coping strategies for information reduction range from the overestimation of the current motif, by addressing urgent but unimportant problems, loss of vision on the whole, up to ignoring information that contradict one's own view etc. [6]. Therefore, checklists and consolidated action plans help to preserve the overview and focus on establishing a functional organization.

To cope with this variety of problems from different professional services largely harmonized joint manuals (DV100) exist for leadership across the organizations [17]. First, the establishment of a small but effective personnel management unit is useful, consisting of an executive assistant, a dispatch rider, a driver and corresponding management tools for information gathering, processing and transmission (checklists, maps, office equipment, radio, etc.).

The execution of command tasks, particularly when during large scale disasters a third level Emergency Operations Command (EOC) with divisions and advisors is established needs not to be restricted to a command post on scene. In particular, the tasks of divisions S1, 4 and 6 (see chapter 11; Figure 15) may be relocated to facilities such as Town Hall enjoying appropriate office, conference and IT infrastructure.

Across organizations the tasks of the divisions are structurally harmonized according to the joint manual DV100 up to individual hospital plans [17;22]. Ultimately, this integrated organizational structure by defining its tasks reduces the need for extensive reorganization and communication.

German Incident Command System

Leadership role in terms of Incident Command up to intermediate incidents below the disaster threshold in all federal states of Germany is assigned to the Chief of the local fire department (FD). In the event a local disaster is declared, the latter obligation passes to the council of the district or the mayor of the city (= main administrative officer (HVB))

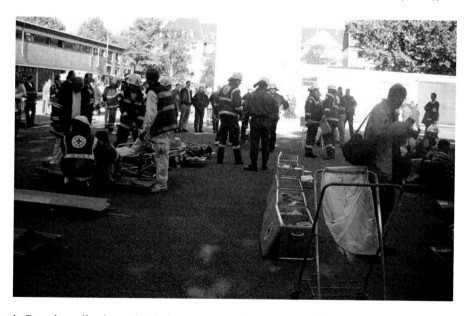

Figure 1. Casualty collecting point during clearance phase organized by DMAT-M: Transport of patients from scene by EMS regarding to priority. Red tag category patients (immediate treatment) right, separated by material boxes form yellow tags (expedited transport) left row. Green tags (minor injury) consolidated care in building background left.

The Chief of FD is, thus, not just commanding all deployed fire brigades, but also the other auxiliary and subordinate organizations. This also applies to EMS Command consisting of Chief FCCS Physician and the EMS organizational leader, but explicitly not in terms of medical measures [9;23], from which a potential for conflict can arise. In practice problems evolve from imprecise definitions of tasks and competencies or incompatible structures of various organizations, especially if the members do not know each other personally. Accordingly, the expected interfaces for the cooperation of different organizations have to take appropriate measures to work effectively [13]. This task is primarily to be accomplished by the section heads and liaison officers, in particular through the establishment of a situation adapted unified command [17]. The tasks of a unified command are to identify the roles and responsibilities, to define measures, to perform situation meetings, to document voting, decision on the nature and extent of warnings, and implementation of public relations.

Subsidiary Leadership in MCI

In general issuing orders to section chiefs and branch leaders in MCI is restricted to definition of missions goals, without strict regulation of means and how to achieve the objectives [1]. Thus incident command allows subordinates freedom of action in implementing goal oriented measures, which is further termed "subsidiary" leadership. In this regard it should be highlighted that it is sought for pragmatic reasons to implement solutions on the lowest appropriate level. However, this type of leadership may not be mixed up with laissez-faire leadership, because the achievement is yet reviewed. In addition, the inferiors in this way are more involved into the overall concept and identify themselves better with their activities. As already mentioned the current leadership approach is based on fractal but centrally controlled organization [2]. Feedback and coordination of objectives is accomplished through the section level along the chain of command. The advantage of this modular organization with small units is the flexible employment of individual components compared to the large Disaster Medical Assistance units during the cold war, which tried to put their rigid organizational structure over each situation.

CHARACTERISTICS OF HIGH-RISK ORGANIZATIONS (HROS)

Built up of spontaneous casualty collecting points (CCP) formed by victims themselves in the initial phase of the mission are, if at all, under very limited control. Therefore, incident command must build upon them, even if they do not meet advanced tactical demands.

To optimize the performance of CCPs and implement long term tactical goals in an early phase FCCS personnel must be assigned to initiate appropriate measures. The latter CCP unit leaders fundamentally decide on the management of space and forces on the spot and further needs to be covered. Thereby they support the deployed EMS staff in organizational terms comparable to the organizational leader at the level of operational command. Through this subsidiary management structure, the operational information deficit is minimized by minimizing misleading communication [1]. Accordingly, measures and solutions are implemented in time with respect to both, the global strategy and the local environment without vertical communication effort. If, however, a vertical communication along the chain of command turns out to be necessary, certain levels of management may not be skipped (DV

100 Section 3.2.4). When urgency demands the latter, the skipped level of command immediately has to be informed [1].

This certain ability of high-risk organizations to detect carefully slight changes in the environment and to react highly flexible through the position holding highest know-how within the HRO has been pointed out by Weick to be characteristic [3]. In contrast, Weick denies the ability of usual business management to communicate errors to decision makers at all, which alone is explained by steep hierarchy and a liability to simplify mental models [4]. This high sensitivity of HROs will, however, be bought with lower specificity, usually leading to false alarms. To prevent overlooking important problems that can escalate, such false alarms must nevertheless be accepted, and, on the opposite, may represent a quality indicator of the vigilance of the system. *"The hallmark of a HRO is not that no errors occur, but that they are not paralyzed by these errors. Flexibility is a mixture of the ability to detect errors early, and the ability by improvised methods to keep on running."* [3] A top management being shielded of bad news, is not in a position to make correct decisions. Due to the complexity of large-scale incident the subsidiary management style on sub-section level is well suited for the achievement of strategic goals which, likewise has been found true in the leadership organization on aircraft carriers at sea [2]. In this regard the human control span of 3-5 downstream sections per sub- section executive must not be exceeded [5;6].

CONCLUSION

As in modern business management the organizational structure in MCIs must follow the process which itself is determined by strategy. To assure proper implementation of strategy the communication structure has lastly to emulate the chain of command, and, by this means limits communication to those forces who *must* exchange information with each other.

In practice, problems occur by imprecise definitions of tasks and competences or from incompatible structures of the various organizations, in particular if the members are not personally acquainted. Therefore, checklists and consolidated disaster preparedness plans help to preserve the overview. In this regard a unified management culture across all Emergency management organizations and agencies is must be assured by a joint leadership manual e.g., DV100 focusing on the establishing a functional global organization.

The primary goal is to be prepared for the important and urgent tasks by reducing tactical communication to a minimum by implementing organizational structure and subsidiary leadership.

REFERENCES

[1]   Kaspari T. Katastrophenschutz in Gesetzen der Länder - Eine vergleichende Darstellung. Ständige Konferenz für Katastrophenvorsorge und Katastrophenschutz 2000.

[2]   SächsBRKG. Gesetz zur Neuordnung des Brandschutzes, Rettungsdienstes und Katastrophenschutzes im Freistaat Sachsen (SächsBRKG). SächsGVBl 2004 Jun 24;245.

[3]   Adams HA, Mahlke L, Lange C, Flemming A. Medizinisches Rahmenkonzept für die überörtliche Hilfe beim Massenanfall von Verletzten (Ü-MANV). Anaesth Intensivmed 2005;46:215-23.

[4]   Adams HA. Versorgung nach Einsatz von ABC- Kampfmitteln- Grundzüge der präklinischen Gefahrenabwehr. Dtsch Ärztebl 2004;101(13):838-43.

[5]   Ruster V, Schmidt J. Einsatzkonzept ÜMANV- Überörtliche Unterstützung beim Massenanfall von Verletzten. Berufsfeuerwehr Köln und Rheinische Projektgruppe "MANV Überörtlich" 2007;1-36.

[6]   Gasch B. Psychologische Aspekte des Massenanfalls von Verletzten. J Anästh Intensivbeh 2005;12(1):98-102.

[7]   Frank M, Heller AR. Sichtung durch Infrastruktur ersetzen - Wunsch und Wirklichkeit. Dtsch Ärztebl 2006;103(48):A3250.

[8]   Sefrin P, Weidringer JW, Weiss W. Sichtungskategorien und deren Dokumentation. Dtsch Ärztebl 2003;100(31-32):A2057-8.

[9]   Weidringer JW. Katastrophenmedizin - Leitfaden für die ärztliche Versorgung im Katastrophenfall. 3 ed. Berlin: Bundesministerium des Inneren; 2003.

[10] BSI. Richtlinien für die Bewältigung von Schadensereignissen mit einer größeren Anzahl Verletzter oder Kranker (Massenanfall von Verletzten). Bekanntmachung des Bayerischen Staatsministeriums des Inneren 1999 Sep 1;ID4-2252.22-7.

[11] Ellinger K, Denz Ch, Luiz T. Großschadensfälle. In: Madler C, Jauch KW, Werdan K, editors. Das NAW- Buch.München: Urban & Schwarzenberg; 1998. p. 922-35.

[12] Lübbe W. Übliche Rechtfertigung für Triage zweifelhaft. Dtsch Ärztebl 2006;103(37):A2362-8.

[13] Weick KE, Sutcliffe KM. Das Unwerwartete managen. 2 ed. Stuttgart: Cotta; 2007.

[14] Chandler A. Strategy and Structure: Chapters in the history of industrial enterprise. New York: Doubleday; 1962.

[15] Rochlin GI, La Porte T.R., Roberts K.H. The Self-Designing High-Reliability Organization- Aircraft Carrier Flight Operations at Sea. Naval War College Review 1998;51(3).

[16] Elleman BA. Communications at sea - integrating the collective. Waves of hope - The US Navy's Response to the Tsunami in Northern Indonesia.Newport, Rhode Island: Naval War College Press; 2006. p. 69-78.

[17] DV 100. Dienstvorschrift DV 100 - Führung und Leitung im Einsatz. Ständige Konferenz für Katastrophenvorsorge und Katastrophenschutz 2000;1-74.

[18] Van den Bossche P. Minds in teams. Maastricht: Datawyse; 2006.

[19] Lavery G. Effective Disaster Communication. In: Farmer JC, Jimenez EJ, Talmor DS, Zimmerman JL, editors. Fundamentals in Disaster Management.Des Plaines/ IL: Society of Critical Care Medicine; 2003. p. 9-20.

[20] Heller AR. Eine Welle der Solidarität - Hochwasser 2002 am Uniklinikum Dresden. In: Koch T, Heller AR, editors. Jahresbericht 2001/02 der Klinik für Anästhesiologie und Intensivtherapie am Uniklinikum Dresden.Dresden: Uniklinikum; 2003. p. 39-50.

[21] Miller GA. The magic number seven plus / minus two. Psychol Rev 1956;63:81-2.

[22] TÜV Süd Life Service. Struktur Krankenhauseinsatzleitung. Notfallmanagementhandbuch Universitätsklinikum Dresden 2007.

[23] Bittger J. Großunfall und Katastrophe Definition, Grundsatzfragen. In: Bittger J, editor. Großunfälle und Katastrophen Einsatztaktik und Organisation.Stuttgart: Schattauer; 1996. p. 2-16.

In: Dresden Teamwork Concept for Medical...
Editor: Axel R. Heller

ISBN 978-1-60692-307-8
© 2009 Nova Science Publishers, Inc.

Chapter 11

DISASTER MANAGEMENT - THE ELBE FLOOD 2002

Axel R. Heller, Sebastian N. Stehr and Michael P. Müller
Department of Anesthesiology & Critical Care Medicine,
University Hospital Carl Gustav Carus, University of Technology, Dresden, Germany

ABSTRACT

Team Management as described within the previous ten chapters is in particular challenged, during natural disasters. Lessons already learned beyond medical skills in leadership, shared mental models, hospital networks, and risk or quality management by the time of disaster onset will be extremely valuable to all concerned parties. This chapter describes as a kind of a captains log the events between August 11 and August 20, 2002 and organizational backgrounds at the University Hospital of Dresden which experienced the greatest evacuation of hospitals in an area in Germany after WW II. The authors were part of the operations command in these days.

PRELUDE

After a deluge of rainfalls on August 11 and 12, 2002 a regional disaster was declared at the same day at 7:20 p.m. in Dresden, the State Capital of Saxony. The high waters of the River Weisseritz that enters the River Elbe from the South within the municipality of Dresden (Figure 1) flash flooded various upstream villages. A second wave of flooding was expected in the city caused, this time, by the waters of the Elbe when the flooded streams of the Erzgebirge receded. The Elbe separates the urban area of Dresden along a stretch of 8 km into the old part of town on the southern left bank and the new town on the northern right bank. The rivers Elbe and Moldau, its main tributary, caused disastrous flooding upstream in the Czech Republic since August 9, 2002 reaching a historic high in Prague on August 14. The Elbe's floodwaters fed by a number of tributaries of similar high water levels were now surging toward Dresden. In the course of the next few days any predictions about the water levels turned out to be less than precise. As a result, it was not possible to fully assess the situation until the crest of 9.40m (2m normal) was reached on Saturday, August 17 at 7:00 a.m. The city was again expecting major breakdowns and potential damage to the urban infrastructure (electricity, water supply, hospitals, nursing homes, cell phone and landline systems, roads and train connections). In addition, a substantial amount of manpower was needed to protect the many cultural sites and treasures (Semper opera house, Zwinger, Ministries etc.).

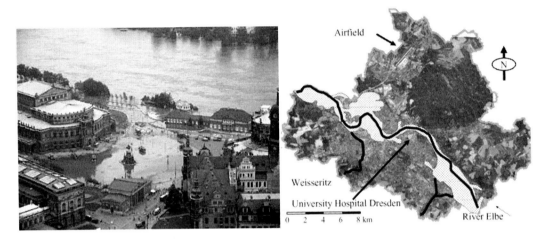

Figure 1. Left: Semper opera house, Theatre Square right: Course of the Elbe in Dresden and flooded areas at water level of 9m (08.16.2002).

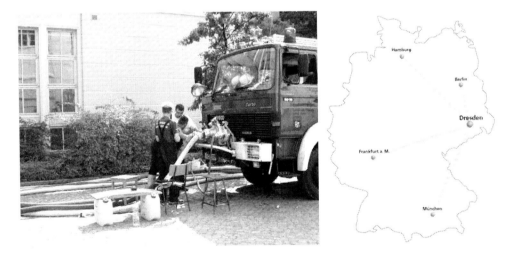

Figure 2. Left: Model LF 16 pump station at building 19, UHD; Fire Dept. Plauen/ Vogtland. Right: Auxiliary Disaster Control Units (medical/ technical/ fire departments) were dispatched from all over Germany. For detailed map of the region see Figure 4 in chapter 9.

MONDAY, 08.12.2002

Around 1:00 p.m. water was breaking into the basements of three buildings of the University Hospital Dresden (UHD). At that time one of the buildings (No. 19, Figure 3) is housing two intensive care units (general/emergency surgery 4th floor and neurosurgery 2nd floor) with a total of 20 respirator-dependant patients. Members of the Dresden fire department started to pump the water out of the basement area. Such incidences of water leakage into these buildings of historic structure do occur in approximately 5-year-intervals under conditions of "normal" flood waters (alert level 2; Figure 14), so that pumping seemed an adequate measure to deal with the problem at that time.

In the course of the afternoon several patients were transferred from the already flooded general hospital of Freital to the ICUs of the UHD. Next day's official forecast for the Elbe water levels is 5.85m-5.95m at 7:00 a.m.

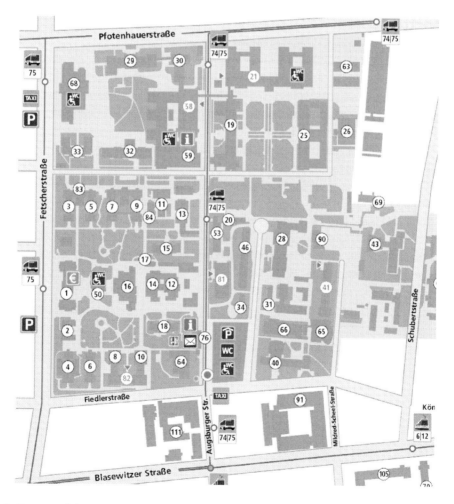

Figure 3. Campus of the University Hospital of Dresden. Core facilities 600 x 500m. North direction at the top of map.

TUESDAY, 08.13.2002

In the early morning hours of August 13 the situation grew more acute when the City Hospital Friedrichstadt (tertiary care hospital) was flash-flooded by the overflowing River Weisseritz and had to evacuate all patients. At the same time the UHD was setting up an operations command to, among other things, deal with accommodation of the 75 patients evacuated from the Friedrichstadt hospital (among those 14 ICU patients). The force was made up as follows: One each medical and administrative representative, chief emergency physician (2 shifts), safety engineer and deputy, legal advisor, crisis center with three telephone lines (internal/external), two to four clerical staff/switch board operators, fax facility, securing direct contact to all chief clinical personnel via phone or pager, briefing room for 20-40 individuals, cartographic material. Team meetings took place every three hours in the operations command center (chief members only). Briefings of the entire staff were carried out twice daily by the medical executive in the lecture hall of the surgical ward until Sunday, August 18.

While the general population is being evacuated from low-lying parts of town around 5:00 p.m. the UHD was given advance warning of an impending disaster. The UHD's geographical location is in the city's East, about 800m south of the river Elbe (at normal water level), yet in a slightly elevated area forming an "island" between the course of the river and the historic riverbed, now the residential area of Dresden-Johannstadt.

Aside from the anesthesiological ICU (new building number 58, classified safe) and the two ICUs mentioned earlier (flooded basements) two additional units are housed on campus in a building of historical structure (No. 4) set up additional facilities for emergency treatment of transfers from other hospitals. As a safety precaution to all those intensive care patients/patients on respirators housed in buildings whose infrastructure (electricity, gas supply) may be jeopardized by rising groundwater levels (some building services and medical engineering are located in basements) all respirator sites were moved to a safe building (central OR number 58). This was accomplished by converting two PACU and ten operating rooms plus induction rooms into ICUs.

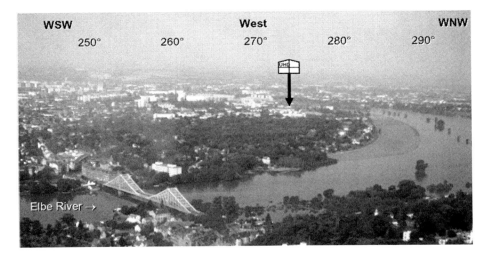

Figure 4. Aerial view of Elbe and UHD (arrow) at water level of 8.9m.

WEDNESDAY/THURSDAY, 08.14/15.2002

Additional relief workers managed to safeguard the electrical system in the hospital's basements against flooding while the Elbe water level stands at 7.0m (alert phase 4). Around 10:00 a.m. the discharge of those patients is started (a good third of a total of 1,200 patients) who are well enough to be released (no medical objections) and have a home to return to. The remaining 800 patients including 80 intensive care patients were efficiently transferred to nationwide hospitals chosen for their capacity to deal with specific serious illnesses. At this point in time the UHD is, within Greater Dresden, the only operational clinical center offering specialized care and has indeed received around 100 patients with such needs from other hospitals. Therefore, an evacuation in the usual sense (scoop and run) did not seem appropriate, all the more since the essential infrastructure and care facilities of the UHD are still safe.

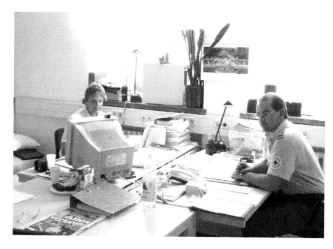

Figure 5. Control center for ambulance service, UHD building 19 (Red Cross Disaster Medical Assistance Team, Wolfratshausen/ Bavaria).

ON SITE LOGISTICS

Under the circumstances it was decided that a "random" transfer, e.g., of ventilated patients to a next available respirator outside the crisis area with no more than a Medical Emergency Triage Tag (METTAG) attached was a potentially risky measure. It was evident that, on principle, disaster medicine and general medicine do not follow the same course of action. Yet both have the same goal, namely the best possible care of all patients under given circumstances. Therefore, the disaster medicine's approach notwithstanding and after weighing local safety aspects it seemed to make more sense, for the time being, to treat ICU patients in the UHD rather than to evacuate at random. If necessary, the physicians in charge (Unified Command and UHD) would have to make individual decisions after weighing risks against benefits, which is the greater risk, to continue full treatment (still possible) in a potentially harmful crisis situation or to transfer to an inadequately equipped hospital, possibly requiring a further transfer with all the logistics involved.

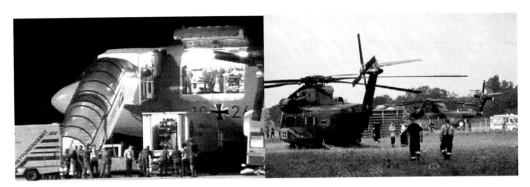

Figure 6. Left : MEDEVAC Airbus A-310/C-160, Armed Forces. Right: Patient transfer in Model CH-53 helicopters from campus (north side non- flooded bank of River Elbe) to airfield.

In decisions like these access to up-to-date information about the current situation was essential. In the evening hours, as water levels continued to rise, it was decided to transfer the remaining patients. In this instance, the involvement of military logistics and infrastructure (MEDEVAC Airbus, CH-53 Helicopter) proved a great advantage because groups of patients could be assembled to be flown to suitable hospitals specializing in maximum and tertiary care while at the same time maintaining their intensive care. This implied, however, that special operational conditions have to be considered such as landing places, flying weather, time of day (especially for CH-53 shuttle flights from hospital to airport), the logistics to be able to load patients on respirators en bloc onto MEDEVAC airbuses (limited oxygen supply on board, limited working hours of the flight crew). The early involvement of a military/tactical consultant proved extremely helpful in this regard.

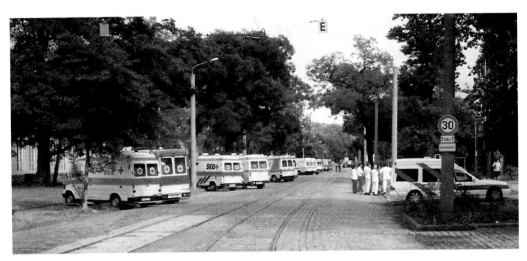

Figure 7. Transportation ready area for nationwide acquired Disaster Medical Assistance Teams, Pfotenhauer Str. northern edge of campus (see also Figure 3).

In liaison with neighboring "safe" hospitals holding enough ICU bed capacity the patients, accompanied by a physician, were transferred by land. The airborne transfer operation "University Hospital Dresden" took place supported by Federal Armed Forces cargo planes (flight of 21 patients on respirators to Leipzig, Berlin, Cologne) during the night of Wednesday, August 14 to Thursday, August 15 and was concluded around 11:00 a.m. on that day. Every ICU patient was accompanied by a member each of the UHD's medical and nursing staff until handed over for further treatment. Those "safe" hospitals on the periphery of the critical area which provide respiratory and treatment facilities and take on patients (not only coming from the UHD) were supported by members of our staff working in shifts until two weeks later (08/28). In its evaluation of the evacuation by the UHD the independent Kirchbach-Commission concludes: "… The process of evacuation turned, ultimately, out to be efficient; the meticulous preparation on part of the University Hospital played a considerable part in it."

On August 14 the regional Bureau of Environment and Geology announced that the floodwater would crest in Dresden on August 15 at 7.50m; the water, however, continued to rise… In the now "empty" UHD where not more than 10 newly treated bone-marrow-transplant recipients whose transfer would have had life-threatening consequences remained in their sterilized bed units, measures to safeguard medical equipment are undertaken on a grand scale. Aside from the tireless work by fire departments and technical relief units from all over the country using 34 Model LF-16 vehicles and pumping 70m^3 of water per minute from the basements, it involved the removal of devices and papers to higher floors. In this regard pumping of water from basements is double edged, because it considerably endangers the structural integrity of a building which may float upward against the elevated groundwater level. Several buildings in town have suffered heavy damage from that mechanism such as the St. Benno High School. Thus, in many instances water free basements were refilled with a layer of sand of a height calculated by a structural engineer, which, again consumed lots of additional manpower. This was impressively demonstrated when two infantry platoons moved into the campus to stabilize the statics of the Heart Center Dresden. Together with Dresden volunteers in hours of back breaking work they carried sand into the basements of the building (Figure 8 left).

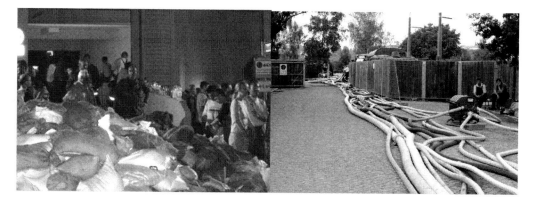

Figure 8. Left: Armed forces together with Dresden volunteers carry sand into the subterranean garage of the Heart Center Dresden. Right: Pumping water on hospital premises (north side) Fire Depts. Kiel & Heide/ Northern- seaside Germany.

Repeatedly the city was hit by power shortages because up to three of four power stations occasionally suffered simultaneous breakdowns. The hospital's emergency-power supply stayed operational.

FRIDAY, 08.16.2002
(WATER LEVEL OF 9.13M AT 10:40 A.M.)

After two waterworks were flooded and the pipe system was contaminated, the drinking water supply to some parts of town was limited. The UHD was not affected; it was checked regularly by the hospital's hygienist. When the power supply to building Nr. 19 could no longer be maintained the hospital's operations command center had to be moved to a safe building (Nr. 66, bone-marrow-transplantation center).

Aside from providing manpower and physical facilities to ensure that ICU capacities in the immediate vicinity of the crisis area were being kept up, starting Friday, August 16 the UHD also supplied shuttle teams consisting of a surgeon, an anesthetist and nursing staff to treat special care cases (neurological, pediatric, thoracic and trauma surgery, gynaecology, urology, ENT, eye clinic) in primary hospitals (Hospitals Dippoldiswalde, Radeberg, and Radebeul, Bavaria-Clinic Kreischa, Joseph-Stift Dresden) as well as in auxiliary hospitals set up on the safe periphery of the flooded area. The course of the Elbe River, however, poses a tactical problem.

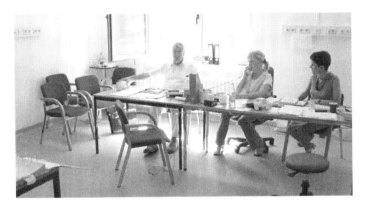

Figure 9. Operations control center, building 66.

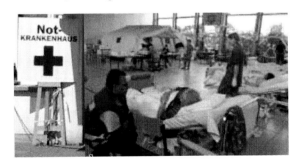

Figure 10. UHD shuttle teams in various primary and auxiliary hospitals: Gym Dresden Plauen High School / run by Johanniter Disaster Medical Assistance Team Hannover.

As a safety precaution some bridges were closed since Thursday, August 15 (water level mark 8,35m at 6:30 p.m.). On Friday, August 16 all of them were closed off so that it became necessary to hold shuttle teams ready on both sides of the river. To be able to reach our team on the right bank via dispatcher (Armed forces/ Federal police Helicopter) in the event of a breakdown in telecommunications, a dispatch center was set up in the building of the Saxon Medical Association (right-bank). An additional auxiliary hospital was staffed and equipped by the UHD on Friday, August 16 in the Fritz-Loeffler High School on the left bank (Dresden-Plauen) and, in co-operation with the Johanniter First Aid Organization, was kept operational until Friday, August 23. It contained the departments of general surgery/trauma surgery, internal medicine, anesthesiology, and intensive care.

In addition to reinforcing local medical care organizations those staff members qualifying as "senior emergency physician" are delegated to the State Capital's operations control center (TEL) on a 24-hour-service for the duration of 8 days. At the same time at least one tactical adviser would be present on each of 4 days. Moreover, aside from the UHD's regular emergency ambulance (Florian DD-81-1) and the helicopter RTH "Christoph 38" additional rescue vehicles were staffed with medical personnel. These vehicles include the Armed Forces helicopter SAR 87 (LTG 62, Holzdorf, stationed at Dresden Airport) equipped with a cable winch, which from August 17 to August 28 was staffed by members of the anesthesiological department, as well as from August 18 to August 21 a secondary helicopter "Elbe-Helicopter 2" (stationed at Bautzen). Given the dramatic situation in the upstream community of Pirna, we staffed a second emergency ambulance in that city.

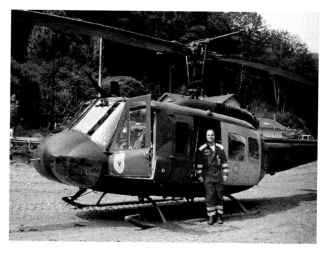

Figure 11. SAR 87, Armed Forces Air Transport Squadron 62, Holzdorf (Model Bell UH-1D) staffed with physicians from UHD anesthesiology department (picture author MPM), 08/17-08/28/2002.

Battery-supplied respirators Models Oxylog (2) and Sulla (7) as well as intensive care respirators Models Servo 900 D (3), Servo 300 (1), and Evita 2 (1) plus the necessary compressed gas cylinders were taken from the anesthesiological units and prepared for pick-up. They had to be stored in a location that was both flood-safe and easily accessible from outside by truck allowing fast and efficient loading (ramps). The outpatients' waiting area in building Nr. 19 met those criteria. Without red tape external auxiliary medical care units continue to get supplied with medication by the hospital's chief emergency physician in close co-operation with the hospital's pharmacy.

SATURDAY, 08.17.2002
(HIGHEST WATER LEVEL OF 9,40M AT 7:00 A.M.)

After intensive preparations, and passing the surveyor's inspection, after the electricity supply to building 58 was secured by employing an external Model 175 KVA emergency-power generator and after getting the official go-ahead to run the facility as a hospital, the unified command was informed at 6:00 p.m., while water levels continue to fall (9.29m), that the UHD will resume ambulatory and stationary health care services for the general public (starting with 100 beds, safe new building 81) in all medical specialties. This closes a gap in the supply of specialized medical service that had existed in the crisis area since August 15 and was bridged only by our shuttle teams working from outside the hospital.

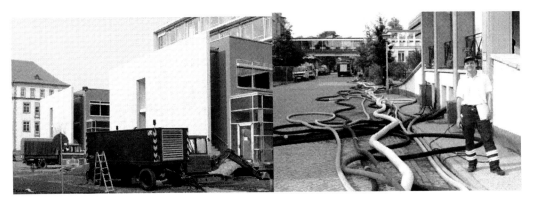

Figure 12. Left: Emergency-power generator Model 175 kVA, Technical Relief Agency (THW), outside building 58. Right Sunday, 08.18.2002, organizational "normality" for chief emergency physician Author ARH, within the disaster.

SUNDAY, 08.18.2002 UNTIL TUESDAY, 08.20.2002

With dropping water levels (Sunday 08/18 7:00 a.m.: 8.90m) the hospital's capacities are gradually expanded and fully restored (100%) by Tuesday, August 20. (level 7:00 a.m.: 6.34m)

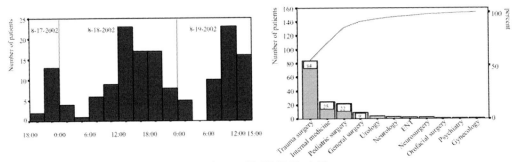

Figure 13. Patient load after restoring service on 08.17.2002, 6:00p.m.

EPILOGUE

The flood water of August 2002 was Saxony's greatest documented natural disaster. It was caused by a series of low pressure systems carrying torrential rainfalls to an area extending from Southern Bohemia to all over Saxony. In the center was the Elbe River catchment's area in the Eastern Erzgebirge suffering unprecedented amounts of rain, up to 406 liter/m²/d on August 12, 2002 approaching the physical maximum. As a result, within the following two days it came to a gradual breakdown of the entire in-patient care in Greater Dresden. 2321 patients had to be evacuated from hospitals and 1286 individuals from nursing homes. The situation was unprecedented for Germany, for which no previous experience could be resorted to. As early as in the afternoon of August 12 the Dresden fire department had established an unified command center (TEL). According to the flood report by the independent commission of the State of Saxony the multitude of simultaneously occurring crisis situations demanded the utmost from the emergency task force and TEL.

Unlike in previous events causing major damage, there was in fact no increase in the number of injuries incurred. On the contrary, it appeared that due to the many flooded traffic routes corresponding road accidents failed to happen so that, in this regard, the hospital's reduced in-care capacities turned out to be less of a problem than expected. But it was the flooding of roads (and the closure of bridges) that posed a particular challenge for the evacuation and shuttle teams as they had to cope with extensive detours and long driving hours. With regard to this problem especially; the use of helicopters (Armed Forces, Border Police, Police) proved invaluable.

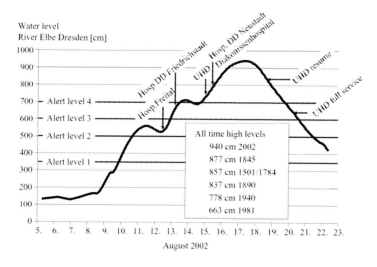

Figure 14. Elbe water levels in August 2002 and blackout of medical services in the Dresden area. Hospitals Freital, Dresden Neustadt, and Dresden Diakonissenkrankenhaus are level 1 centers. The Dresden Friedrichstadt Hospital and University Hospital Dresden (UHD) are tertiary care centers.

Although auxiliary hospitals (a total of three) had been set up to meet an increased demand in care facilities, medical treatment on-site could – despite all good intentions - at best comply with that of an out-patient hospital. Both, patient load and "bed occupancy" as well as appropriate requests for help to the UHD by colleagues working in those places were evidence for this fact. Sanctioned by the unified command, the UHD provided assistance within available means. Consequently, what all efforts had to aim for was to restore the UHD's operational capability as fast as possible, in order to be able to provide the maximum care of a fully equipped hospital. Urgent surgery, e.g., cesarean sections, under risky field conditions that would have involved a great amount of expense and commitment of a considerable number of external resources had to be avoided.

Just like logistic structures are challenged in an extreme situation as this, professional and personal relations are tested. Those who were a part of it got to know each other better. Interpersonal relations were mostly positive; but there were negative experiences as well. Lessons have to be learned from those days' events and should be consistently applied, so that procedures can be carried out more precisely and promptly in the future. The system has to be professionally structured and not have to depend on the improvisational skills of individuals. Even at hospital level, this includes clear disaster control instructions and channels of communication that insure the essential feed-back and avoid wasting time.

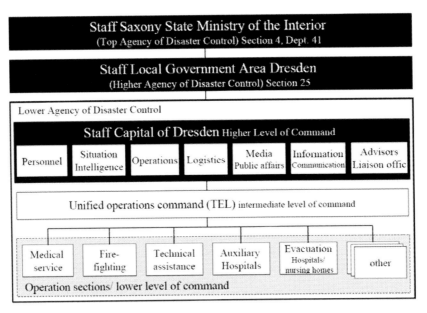

Figure 15. Management levels and disaster control organization during flood, Dresden 2002.

All those involved (inside and outside) should be informed promptly about who is responsible for what. Implementation of the joint leadership manual (DV100) harmonized across safety organizations was one of the lessons learned. For Three-hourly staff meetings (10-20 participants) and the once or twice daily briefing for all co-workers present on campus proved to be helpful. Moreover, the measure of having UHD's senior emergency physicians both onsite and at the same time at TEL has definitely proved itself, because they both were familiar with the inner structure of the hospital (infrastructure/personnel) making any communication between TEL and hospital more effective. The problem of interfacing, that can be quite stultifying, is thus eliminated. However, the necessary telecommunications and personnel structures - requirements for a prompt exchange of information particularly at TEL – have to be available.

ACKNOWLEDGEMENTS

At this point we would, again, like to thank all of the relief workers of the disaster control agencies (Fire Departments, Disaster Medical Assistance Teams, Technical Relief Agency, Armed Forces etc.) nationwide as well as the Dresden volunteers and all colleagues for their untiring commitment. In the face of this national catastrophe all helpers showed enormous motivation and drive. They had to endure restraints on all areas of their daily lives, as for example having to catch some sleep with the constant noise of engines running. Also, the generous support by the neighboring hospitals and clinics contributed to the fact that we were able to give optimum care to our patients outside the UHD. We all, collectively, managed to evacuate our patients safely and to restore the hospital's operational capability for the greater good of the people of the region. It was particularly awe-inspiring to witness the degree of solidarity among all those involved in the cause that brought us together as one team in those days.

REFERENCES

[1]   Adams HA, Mahlke L, Lange C, Flemming A. Medizinisches Rahmenkonzept für die überörtliche Hilfe beim Massenanfall von Verletzten (Ü-MANV). Anaesth Intensivmed 2005;46:215-23.

[2]   Albrecht DM: Bilder die bleiben. Carus Intern, Sonderausgabe August 2002

[3]   Bittger J. Kommunikationsmanagement bei Großschadenslagen und Katastrophen. In: Bittger J, Ed. Großunfälle und Katastrophen Einsatztaktik und Organisation .Stuttgart: Schattauer; 1996. p. 94-110.

[4]   Bittger J: Großunfall und Katastrophe In: Bittger J (Ed.) Großunfälle und Katastrophen Einsatztaktik und –organisation. Schattauer 1996: 1-16

[5]   Burger R: Die Flughafenklinik – Nach der größten Krankenhausevakuierung in der Nachkriegsgeschichte. Frankfurter Allgemeine Zeitung 22.08.2002 Nr. 194, S8

[6]   DIVI/ IAG Schock. Stellungnahme der Interdisziplinäre Arbeitsgruppe (IAG) Schock der Deutschen Interdisziplinären Vereinigung für Intensivmedizin und Notfallmedizin (DIVI) zur Patientenversorgung im Katastrophenfall. Anaesth Intensivmed 2006;47(451):454.

[7]   Elleman BA. Communications at sea - integrating the collective. Waves of hope - The US Navy´s Response to the Tsunami in Northern Indonesia.Newport, Rhode Island: Naval War College Press; 2006. p. 69-78.

[8]   Frank M, Heller AR. Sichtung durch Infrastruktur ersetzen - Wunsch und Wirklichkeit. Dtsch Ärztebl 2006;103(48):A3250.

[9]   Gasch B. Psychologische Aspekte des Massenanfalls von Verletzten. J Anästh Intensivbeh 2005;12(1):98-102.

[10] Jäger B. Führungsstrukturen bei aufgabenübergreifenden Einsätzen von Feuerwehr, Rettungsdienst und Polizei am Beispiel des Landes Hessen. Wiesbaden, Gießen: Verwaltungsfachhochschule - Fachbereich Polizei -; 2007.

[11] Kirchbach HP: Bericht der unabhängigen Kommission der sächsischen Staatsregierung zur Flutkatastrophe 2002. Internet site: www.sachsen.de/de/bf/ hochwasser/programme/ download/Kirchbach_Bericht.pdf

[12] Lavery G. Effective Disaster Communication. In: Farmer JC, Jimenez EJ, Talmor DS, Zimmerman JL, editors. Fundamentals in Disaster Management.Des Plaines/ IL: Society of Critical Care Medicine; 2003. p. 9-20.

[13] Miller GA. The magic number seven plus / minus two. Psychol Rev 1956;63:81-2.

[14] Möhring C: Leid bringt zusammen – Hunderte von Patienten wurden aus Dresdner Kliniken in andere Krankenhäuser gebracht. Frankfurter Allgemeine Zeitung 16.08.2002 Nr. 189, S9

[15] Rochlin GI, La Porte T.R., Roberts K.H. The Self-Designing High-Reliability Organization- Aircraft Carrier Flight Operations at Sea. Naval War College Review 1998;51(3).

[16] Seliger K. Rapid Response - Notfallmanagement und behördenübergreifende Zusammenarbeit. In: Industry Solution Sales Public Germany, editor. IBM Software Group; 2007. p. 1-17.

[17] Shapira SC, Shemer J. Medical Management of Terrorist Attacks. In: Shemer J, Shoenfeld Y, editors. Terror and medicine.Lengerich: Pabst Science Publishers; 2003. p. 50.

[18] Stein M, Hirshberg A. Limited Mass casulties due to Conventional Weapons - The daily Reality of a Level 1 Trauma Center. In: Shemer J, Shoenfeld Y, editors. Terror and medicine.Lengerich: Pabst Science Publishers; 2003. p. 378-93.

[19] Strauss H, Schüttler J: Katastrophenmanagement im Krankenhaus: Empfehlungen für den Ärztlichen Dienst. In: German ministry of the Interior (Eds.) Katastrophenmedizin-Leitfaden für die ärztliche Versorgung im Katastrophenfall 2. Aufl. 2002, 227-241

[20] Taylor JL, Roup BJ, Blythe D, Reed GK, Tate TA, Moore KA. Pandemic Influenza Preparedness in Maryland: Improving Readiness Through a Tabletop Exercise. Biosecurity and Bioterrorism 2005;3(1):61-9.

[21] Töpfer A. Krisenverlaufs-Matrix: Verzahnung von Krisenmanagement und Krisenkommunikation. In: Töpfer A, editor. Die A-Klasse: Elchtest, Krisenmanagement, Kommunikationsstrategie.Neuwied: Luchterhand; 1999. p. 143-53.

[22] TÜV Süd Life Service. Struktur Krankenhauseinsatzleitung. Notfallmanagementhandbuch Universitätsklinikum Dresden 2007.

[23] Van den Bossche P. Minds in teams. Maastricht: Datawyse; 2006.

[24] Weick KE, Sutcliffe KM. Management of the unexpected. 2 ed. Stuttgart: Cotta; 2007.

[25] Weidringer JW: Aspekte zur Katastrophenmedizin und Definition ihrer Inhalte und Aufgaben. In: Bundesministerium des Inneren (Hrsg.) Katastrophenmedizin- Leitfaden für die ärztliche Versorgung im Katastrophenfall 2. Aufl. 2002, 25-28

INDEX

F

G

J

L

M

N

Q

R

U

V

W